PHYSICAL THERAPY LEADERSHIP BOOK

LEADERSHIP IN PRIVATE PRACTICE

WHAT IT TAKES TO BECOME A WORLD CLASS LEADER AND CEO OF A SUCCESSFUL PRIVATE PRACTICE

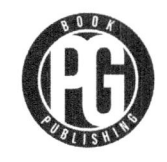

PAUL GOUGH

Paul Gough Publishing

Copyright © 2020 Paul Gough. All rights reserved.

This publication is licensed to the individual reader only. Duplication or distribution by any means, including email, disk, photocopy, and recording, to a person other than the original purchaser, is a violation of international copyright law.

Publisher: Paul Gough, 25 Raby Road, Hartlepool, UK, TS24 8AS

While they have made every effort to verify the information here, neither the author nor the publisher assumes any responsibility for errors in, omissions from or a different interpretation of the subject matter. This information may be subject to varying laws and practices in different areas, states, and countries. The reader assumes all responsibility for the use of the information.

The author and publisher shall in no event be held liable to any party for any damages arising directly or indirectly from any use of this material. Every effort has been made to accurately represent this product and its potential and there is no guarantee that you will earn any money using these techniques.

ISBN: 9798697264379

ALSO BY PAUL GOUGH:

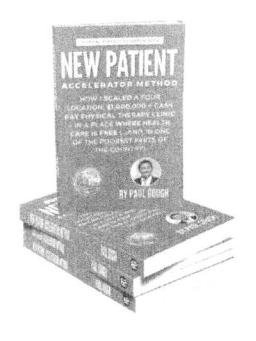

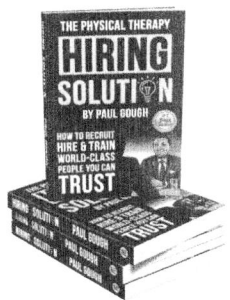

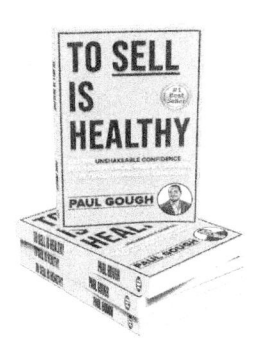

New Patient Accelerator Method:
"How I Scaled a Four Location, $1,000,000 + Cash Pay Physical Therapy Clinic - In a Place Where Health Care Is Free (...And, in One of the Poorest Areas of the Country)"
www.PaulsMarketingBook.com

The Physical Therapy Hiring Solution:
"How to Recruit, Hire and Train World-Class People You Can Trust"
www.PaulsHiringBook.com

To Sell Is Healthy:
"Get The Unshakeable Confidence to Sell Your Physical Therapy Services – At Twice The Price You Are Now"
www.PaulsHiringBook.com

The Healthy Habit:
"Learn Secrets To Keep Active, Maintain Independence And Live Free From Painkillers. Essential Reading For People Aged 50+"
www.PaulsHealthyHabit.com

DEDICATION

This book is dedicated to my Grandma Rose.

She was, and remains, the ultimate example to me of what is required of a great family leader. She sat at the head of my mother's side of the family for 86 years and provided us all with every ounce of support, challenge, attention and guidance that we each needed – anytime we needed it. She showed me what real courage looks like and what it takes to raise a family that is bound together by its values and sticks to its principles.

I was lucky to have my Grandma live across the road from the school I went to so it meant I could leave school and get an amazing lunch or dinner cooked for me, any day I liked. And I can tell you I really did make the most of that privilege. Best, that tradition continued on for many years into my adult life and sitting down at the dinner table with my Grandma (and Grandad) is to this day STILL one of the best and most cherished experiences of my life.

As the eldest Grandson, I was blessed to have my Grandma in my life for 38 years and I can honestly say I loved every second of every minute I got to spend with her. Grandma's house was always a special place to be and I never felt safer, more comfortable, made to feel special and more loved than when I was with her (and my Grandad) sat on the sofa in their home.

**I am eternally grateful and blessed.
Thanks Grandma. I love you.**

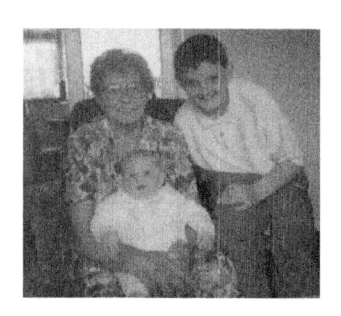

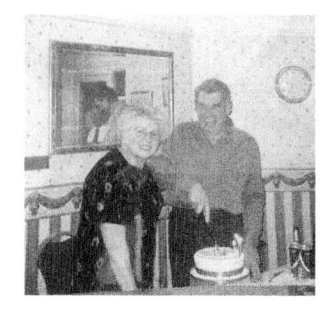

GET YOUR FREE RESOURCE KIT: PAULGOUGH.COM/LEADERSHIP-RESOURCE

BEFORE YOU READ THE BOOK GET YOUR LEADERSHIP BOOK FREE RESOURCE KIT

To support you on your journey of becoming a better Leader and CEO of your private practice, I have some very important resources that I want you to have for FREE:

Go To: www.paulgough.com/leadership-resource to get them.

When you do, here's what you will receive:

- **CEO Job Description and Scorecard** – how can you do the job properly if you don't know what the job requires? This CEO job description and scorecard is there to act as your guide to ensure that you're doing ONLY the work required of a CEO (you will need to have this in your hand before getting to part 2 of the book)

- **Strategic Growth Plan Template** – this is a "fill in the blanks" style template with instructions on how to create your practice growth plan (which, as you will discover from the CEO score card document, is one of your most important jobs)

- **Pauls leadership Philosophy Template** – this is a copy of the document that I created to give to my team which outlines and explains my own leadership style philosophy. Basically, it is a way of telling new staff how they can expect to be managed by me when they come and work for me. It's there to prompt your own ideas and stimulates your thoughts so you create your own

- **Company Organizational Chart Examples PDF** – structure brings freedom. Function follows form. If you don't have the right company structure your company can't grow effectively. This is an example of how your company structure could look

- **Masterclass 1 (Video): "Understanding the Role of a Top CEO"** – in this instant download video you will discover the 7 most critical aspects of running a private practice without being tied to it every day. The video is LIVE from stage in Orlando where I am teaching a room full of private practice owners like you on the topic of business leadership

- **Masterclass 2 (Video): "Leadership: How to Inspire Lasting Change in Your People"** – this is another instant download video for you to watch. This one was recorded LIVE from stage in New Orleans where I was talking about leadership and what it really takes to bring about change in your organization

To get the best out of this book, and to give yourself an advantage over other private practice owners, get all of your CEO resources now:

www.paulgough.com/leadership-resource

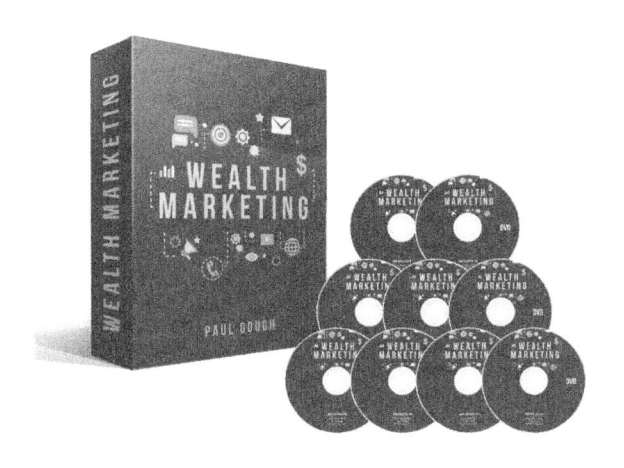

GET YOUR FREE WEALTH MARKETING GIFT FROM PAUL, NOW...

Go to: **www.paulgough.com/wealth-gift**
To get this instant access 9 DVD video program, NOW.

**Claim your $1,997.00 worth of cash patient generating, higher profit making, wealth marketing DVD program,
absolutely FREE!**

Including a FREE "Test-Drive" of Paul Gough's Cash Club Membership that sends to your clinic $10,000 worth of marketing ideas every 30 days.

**Claim your copy now, at
www.paulgough.com/wealth-gift**

GET YOUR FREE RESOURCE KIT: PAULGOUGH.COM/LEADERSHIP-RESOURCE

PRAISE FOR PAUL GOUGH FROM PHYSICAL THERAPISTS ALL OVER THE WORLD

. . . .

"Paul has helped me develop and lead a team of people to help me to see the blind spots in my business that I was too close to see. Thanks to Paul's CEO Mastermind program, I now have confidence that I am making the best next decisions in my business."
Kevin Vandi, Competitive EDGE Physical Therapy, San Jose

"Working with Paul has helped me to make substantial growth as a business owner, scale our business, and I've been able to safely remove myself from the day-to-day operations that would otherwise keep me stuck!"
Payal Patel, Adapt Physical Therapy, NJ

"Paul has helped me to grow and scale a real business that is now able to run without me. I love the tight knit group of like-minded colleagues who have become my biggest supporters and confidants. Paul's CEO Mastermind group has helped me sort out problems in the best and most efficient way possible."
Carrie Jose, CJ Physical Therapy and Pilates, NH

"The biggest benefit of working with Paul's CEO Mastermind is having the opportunity to be in a room with other top business owners who are able to expand the calibre of your thinking. The people in your group have no emotional attachment to your business and they are able to help you see blind spots and provide advice from points of view you can't see. Equally important, you receive the guidance, support and accountability to help you make better decisions ensuring your business moves forward and in the right direction."
Oscar Andalon, LEVEL4 PT & Wellness, CA

"If you are at the point in your business where it is stagnant and you're not sure which direction to go in to make it more profitable, this CEO Mastermind group is, in my opinion, what is needed."
Hooman Javanmardi, Prime Therapy and Pain Center, CA

GET YOUR FREE RESOURCE KIT: PAULGOUGH.COM/LEADERSHIP-RESOURCE

"Working closely with Paul has been the best business decision I have ever made. Now I have clarity all year long".
Christine Astarita, Breakthrough Intensive Physical Therapy, NY

"Being a part of Paul's coaching group is like having a board of directors that are invested in the success of your business. You have access to business owners with different perspectives to provide guidance for growth and problem solving which helps curb owner bias towards making emotional decisions - which are rarely ever the right ones."
John Salva, Impact Physio, PA

"Working with Paul has given me invaluable clarity on what my focus should be for my business and what adjustments I need to make – which are never the ones I thought they would be!"
Jonathan Ruzicka, RPM Physical Therapy, TX

"If you are confused about what has your business stuck and not growing to the potential that you want, working with Paul helps you identify the REAL problems/opportunities that you need to change to see huge gains."
Paul Hendricks, Body Balance Physical Therapy Lakeway, TX

GET YOUR FREE RESOURCE KIT: PAULGOUGH.COM/LEADERSHIP-RESOURCE

X   @THEPAULGOUGH

GET YOUR FREE RESOURCE KIT: PAULGOUGH.COM/LEADERSHIP-RESOURCE

CONTENTS

CHAPTER 1

Could Everything You've Ever Been Told About Leadership Be Wrong? - 27

CHAPTER 2

What's the Difference Between A Manager And Leader? - 43

CHAPTER 3

It's All About the People - 61

CHAPTER 4

How to Inspire Lasting Change In Your People - 77

CHAPTER 5

Liberate, Don't Abdicate – 87

CHAPTER 6

What Are the Qualities of Great Leaders? – 107

CHAPTER 7
Developing Your Own Leadership Philosophy – 131

CHAPTER 8
What Phase of Business Ownership Are You In? – 151

CHAPTER 9
Create the Growth Plan - 171

CHAPTER 10
Understanding the Numbers and Developing Financial Clarity- 195

CHAPTER 11
Recruit A Players and Build The Team – 211

CHAPTER 12
Retain and Coach A Players – 233

CHAPTER 13
Developing A Great Culture – 255

CHAPTER 14
Avoid the Number One Reason Businesses Fail – 273

GET YOUR FREE RESOURCE KIT: PAULGOUGH.COM/LEADERSHIP-RESOURCE

INTRODUCTION:
PAINT THE FENCE – OR WRITE A BOOK?

I will forever refer to this as my "lockdown book." That is because I wrote this book during the six weeks that I was locked down in my home in Florida during the COVID-19 pandemic. Although unexpected, and obviously not the situation I wanted to be in, I chose to see lockdown as an *opportunity* to do something that would add significant value to my life.

Lockdown presented me with a choice: I could sit by my pool and soak up the Florida sunshine, paint my fence, or search online for a new kitchen that the house didn't need. Or I could use the time that I'd found – with not being able to go places or do things that I ordinarily would have done – to write this book.

I made the decision to **prioritize** this book.

I used the skills that I've learned from running my businesses to look critically at what lockdown really meant to me. I considered all of the things the government stopped me from doing and to my surprise and delight, I worked out that I was set to be given an extra 10 to 12 hours per week in my life.

They say that there's no way to add more hours to the day – but it appeared to me that through lockdown I found just that.

I was unable to drive to work each day, I couldn't go to watch the kids at soccer, and I couldn't even hang out with Natalie in a restaurant.

The coffee shop near my home remained open during lockdown for takeout, but it was very quiet. That saved me another ten minutes every day by not having to wait in line. Heck, I calculated that I would save

GET YOUR FREE RESOURCE KIT: PAULGOUGH.COM/LEADERSHIP-RESOURCE

around ten more minutes every day by not having to pack the kids and all of their stuff in and out of the car.

In total, just these few things alone – not driving to work, not waiting in line for a coffee and not packing the kids into the car every morning - would save me a total of thirty minutes per day. Thirty minutes?

Doesn't sound a lot, right?

Maybe not.

But that same thirty minutes equates to about 750 words written in this book every day.

Yes, you really are reading this book today simply because of that thirty minutes that was given to me during lockdown.

Things were taken away, but extra time was coming into my life and I had a *choice* about how I would use that time.

Would I spend it or invest it?

Sure, a fresh lick of paint on the garden fence would have made it look nicer – but would it serve to add any real and lasting value to my life? Unlikely.

And yes, I *could* spend more time by the pool – that's always tempting when you live in Florida – but there's only so much of that you can do before it gets monotonous and makes you feel lethargic.

And as for a new kitchen, I honestly couldn't think of anything worse than having to incur the mental torture of picking a red door over a black door or a wooden work top over a granite one. Not to mention that it would only kickstart a series of other "improvements" to the home that weren't needed, but that Natalie would most likely want simply because the kitchen was new and now everything else looked old (ever noticed how that always seems to happen?).

Amazon seemed to keep a lot of people busy through lockdown, so I guess I could have spent some time on there?

But other than to buy books, I think I've used it about twice in my life and I can't even recall what I bought. I've heard it's called the "Everything Store," and I would agree. It's the ability to buy everything that I don't need and only ever would if I was bored or unfulfilled. It has the cheapest prices on everything that I can live without or that I don't need in the first place.

These things are examples of the thousands of distractions vying for your time and attention. They're designed to keep you busy. You could say they are the <u>choice you make when you don't want to do the things that will actually make a real and lasting difference to your life</u>.

They're also the types of distractions that show up in your private practice every day.

Whether it is the latest drama happening with your front desk, yet another billing issue, a member of your staff not showing up for work (again), patients not re-booking or dropping off the schedule – all of these things are examples of the stuff that so often consumes a practice owner's time. It's how you end up tired and yet what you wanted was to make money and have more free time.

As a business owner, constantly getting involved in these types of distractions **isn't** the best use of your time. It's what's keeping you stuck at the level you are. It's why there's a lot of activity in your life but little in the way of accomplishment. It's why you're moving – but there's not much momentum.

What is more, if you are always getting caught up in these types of distractions, it's also a clear sign that you've got other, more deep-rooted problems that you need to get to the bottom of. Massaging a tight

GET YOUR FREE RESOURCE KIT: PAULGOUGH.COM/LEADERSHIP-RESOURCE

hamstring doesn't do much if you've got a problem at the sciatic nerve. Painkillers don't do much if you've got a brain tumour.

TIME IS THE GREATEST DEMOCRACY ON EARTH

If you're always fixing problems or fighting fires, chances are the *real* issue is that you're prioritizing your time and focusing your activities **on the wrong things.** You're busy – but not productive. You're working hard – but on the wrong things.

I believe time is the greatest democracy. Perhaps the only *true* democracy on Earth? Each one of us has the same amount of time available. What we do with it is ultimately what dictates the outcomes and success we get. And what you're about to learn is that, as a CEO of a private practice, you have a choice on how you use your time.

You can *spend* time – or you can *invest* it.

If you're saying "yes" to something that is instantly gratifying – like painting the fence – then you're saying "no" to something else (like writing a book.)

If you're saying "yes" to always fixing the dramas in your practice, you're saying "no" to changing the recruitment process that would solve the problem once and for all.

If you're saying "yes" to doing more social media – even though it isn't working in the first place – you're likely saying "no" to allocating time for creating a comprehensive and robust marketing plan that would include at least six other ways of bringing in more patients, reducing your reliance on social media in the first place.

If you're saying "yes" to always having to fight with your team when they keep screwing up the billing in your clinic, you're saying "no" to training those people and creating a process that is fool proof.

Time is like money. If you spend it, it is gone.

However, if you invest it properly – on things that will free up your time – it's wholly possible to put yourself in a situation where you're achieving more, getting more stuff done, experiencing more success, and at the same time, feeling like you've got more time on your hands.

Despite what most people think, there really isn't any correlation between doing more work and achieving more success. There is, however, a direct correlation between what you choose to do – prioritize – and the success you enjoy.

This is an important first lesson – perhaps the most important in all of this book. A CEO's *time* is the most valuable of all assets. How you use your time largely dictates the success of your practice and the quality of your life choices.

It's 100 percent possible to do the right thing at the wrong time. And many do. That is why you've got to become world-class at prioritizing your time and activities. It is the ultimate skill that you need to be a great business leader.

To do it successfully, you've first got to know what the actual tasks are you should be doing and that requires you to know what the real job of a CEO actually is. That's precisely what we're going to cover in the pages of this book.

In the end, business success comes down to getting the CEO of the company in a position to do the job required of the CEO. If you're always involved in the work that your front desk person should be doing – you're a CEO in name only. You're taking on all of the hassle and responsibility of owning a company and you're getting none of the upside. You're doing $15 per hour work. And if you are, it should come as no surprise to you when at the end of the month all you made was the equivalent of $15 per hour. You made the decision to prioritize $15 per hour work and you were paid accordingly.

Ultimately, everything about your business and how it looks today is determined by the decisions you made yesterday. If your decision making – your prioritizing – was poor, so too will be the results of your business. Another way to look at it, if you want to know how your business will look in the future – just look at the decisions you're making today. Decision making and prioritizing really is that important.

HOW THIS BOOK IS STRUCTURED – THE TWO PARTS

As we work through this book together, I want you to keep this in your mind: Great leaders are great communicators. They can motivate, and they can inspire and rally their troops. We will cover all of that in Part One of this book (You, the Leader). But, as you will find out in Part 2 (You, the CEO), if you can't prioritize your time, and ultimately that of your people, you end up working very hard, but on the wrong things. That's only going to make you tired and it's going to give you very little in the way of rewards.

Think about it like this: What you say "no" to is ultimately what defines the success of your life – not what you said "yes" to.

Throughout lockdown, I said "no" to spending my time on instantly gratifying things (such as painting the fence) and that meant I could say "yes" to writing a book with the additional ten hours I found every week in my life thanks to six weeks of lockdown. Saying "no" to distractions puts you in a position to say "yes" to more of the right things that have lasting impact.

As a result, this book will serve to provide a lifelong, possibly multi-generational, asset that will add significant income and value to my life. It's part of my much bigger strategy for achieving success and fulfilment.

And here's the best part.

Perhaps if I make enough money through sales of this book, I can hire someone else to paint the bloody fence or cut the grass for me next time there might be a lockdown.

Ultimate lesson: a great CEO does not spend time. He or she *invests* it.

A FIELD REPORT - NOT THEORY

As you read this book, you should understand where the ideas, concepts, and principles are coming from. I've spent more than a decade running a private practice that has repeatedly made a six-figure net profit. In recent years, I've left the day-to-day running of the practice to become a "remote CEO."

I run that practice, which is in the UK, from 3,500 miles away in Florida.

I've learned a lot of lessons about what it takes to keep a business making money – even though I'm not there every day. I'll share many of those lessons in this book.

What is more, I now own and run a group of companies that span across two different countries (UK and the United States) and three different fields (medical, media, and property). I've got more than thirty people on my payroll with everyone from a finance director to general and mid-level managers and the combined total revenues of those companies is closer to $5,000,000 than it is $4,000,000.

I've also spent years working with thousands of private practice owners like you. Recently, in my **CEO Mastermind Program**, I've been up close and personal, looking under the hoods of as many as forty businesses every year and coaching those private practice owners on how to become great CEOs so that they can exit the day-to-day running of their own practices.

We sit in a ten-person boardroom-style meeting four times per year and I get to act as the head of their company board.

Each person in the room presents the company's results and explains the challenges as well as the plan they have for further growth.

What is funny is that it nearly always turns out that what the business owner originally *thought* they should be working on was, in fact, the completely wrong thing. They nearly always talk about the symptom and rarely are they able to understand the actual cause (that needs their attention).

In the meeting we aim to highlight what this real cause of the problem is and we get to the bottom of any growth challenges holding the business back. After diagnosing the REAL problem, we send the business owner on his or her way with a plan to execute and the owner leaves confident and assured that what is about to be worked on – where time is about to be invested – is the thing that should be worked on.

When it comes to actually allocating your time and effort, doesn't it help to be sure that what you're about to spend your time and money on is actually the thing you should be?

When you have it confirmed by 10 other people – successful peers you trust and respect who have no hidden agenda other than to want you to be successful – it's much easier to go away and put everything you've got into the plan. No more half-built bridges or great ideas left on the table. And definitely no working hard on the wrong things, constantly spinning your wheels with little if any progress.

In CEO Mastermind, I lead the room, I offer direction and clarity, and as a group we provide a stress test to the plan to ensure that what they're about to work on is the right thing. Every three months, we get back together to review the progress and continue to stress test the plan for the next quarter. On and on it goes. Onwards and upwards the business grows. Better and better the lifestyle of the owner.

Again, much of what I've learned from coaching those business owners is included in this book. Put another way, **this is a field report**. None of what you're about to read is theory. And, as is always the case with my work, you can say you don't like it or that you don't agree with it. *But you can't say it doesn't work.*

PAUL GOUGH'S CEO MASTERMIND PROGRAM

At the end of the book, you'll get to find out more about my **CEO Mastermind Program**. If it's something that you're interested in, be sure to contact my office to find out your suitability.

If you understand and can see the value in coaching – and having a peer group of successful business owners looking at your own business every three months – pointing things out that you may not be able to see – then you will love what the program can do for you.

Simply send an email to paul@paulgough.com with the subject line "CEO Program Interest" to find out how it works.

We've had private practice owners from all over the world join the program and the only condition is that you're employing people and you're planning on growing fast in the next 12-18 months.

Anyhow, let's get into the book. I'm excited to share with you more than a decade's worth of lessons learned and challenges overcome that have helped me to not only make money from my practice, but to also live a terrific life full of real choices and opportunity.

It's hard to have one without the other and what you'll discover is that many of the skills you learn in becoming a great CEO for your practice can also be applied to improve your life. Win-win.

Enjoy the book and be sure to take notes along the way.

Paul.

PART 1:
YOU, THE LEADER

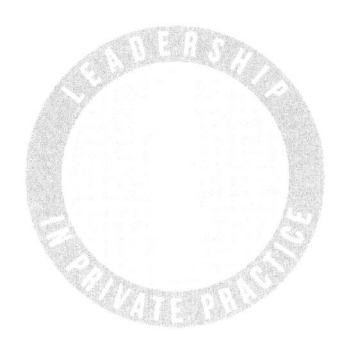

COULD EVERYTHING YOU'VE EVER BEEN TAUGHT ABOUT LEADERSHIP BE WRONG?

The great irony of being a leader and CEO of a private practice is that many who make it to that level have no clue how they even got there. Having focused for so long on providing great medical care to patients, the happy by-product is an increased volume of patients – enough that they can't all be serviced by you alone, which leads to the inevitable forming of an organization known as a company.

This company is now responsible for complex legal and financial notes owed to the government, not to mention the welfare and well-being of a group of people called employees. These are people you agree to pay weeks in advance of the revenue they bring in – regardless of how well your company is doing. At least the government only wants to be paid if you've made some money first.

As well as new legal and personnel obligations, you've still got the ongoing responsibility of providing a high-quality service to your patients.

When it was just you, you could be sure the patient experience was magical. Now that ten other people are involved, all you can do is hope and pray they're all bringing their "A-game." If one doesn't, you'll soon know about it because it will be written up in a Google review for the rest of the world to see.

The very fact that you've had to bring in more employees means that your expenses have gone up. Inevitably, you'll need to raise the fees just to cover the additional costs. Selling "you" at a lower price was easy. Selling someone else at a higher price – that is a different story altogether. A new marketing and sales system are now required, but they don't come cheap and aren't easy to implement when you've got so many other things to consider.

Paying out for employees and spending on marketing requires you to pay close attention to your cash flow. Managing cash is often as difficult as managing people, yet it's nearly always an afterthought. It only becomes a priority when you've run out. Cash is like oxygen to a business. If you don't get enough of it coming in, you'll die very quickly.

As the saying goes, "You can exist for years without profit, but you can't exist a week without cash." Cash is king – and as the owner of a private practice, you have to know how to bring it in faster than it goes out.

If you ask any business owner if they'd ever considered any of these things *before* they'd formed the company, they'd *probably* tell you no. If you asked the same business owner if they'd ever considered how much hassle and heartache would come as a result of these things, they *definitely* tell you no.

GET YOUR FREE RESOURCE KIT: PAULGOUGH.COM/LEADERSHIP-RESOURCE

The problem is this: when you reach the point of realizing how difficult it is to do all of this – lead people, manage cash flow, build a marketing system etc. – while simultaneously trying to keep your sanity and find time for your family, it's often the case that you're past the point of no return. Your proverbial ass is on the line for a costly office space, the line of credit needed to get to this point is secured against your family home, oh, and that's on top of the business startup loan you took out to get your company off the ground in the first place.

Above all, your self-worth is attached to making this thing work by *any* means.

Even though everyone around you tells you not to pursue it, your pig-headedness has you believing that you *will* work it out and that you *will* prove them all wrong, in the end. Your future success will come at any cost, including your health, your sanity, and most definitely time away from your family.

What's more, it is very likely that you'll forgo a decent salary.

You'll be "happy" to earn less than most of your employees, and you'll do it in the hope that, one day, *someday*, this company will pay out and you'll be able to tell everyone that the rewards justified the means. You quite literally mortgage your future on the hope that your company will one day pay dividends.

Welcome to Hell!

Welcome to the loneliest and oftentimes most frustrating and sometimes lowest-paid job on the planet. It's madness, but everything I've just described is so often how it plays out for a small business owner. If you knew back then all of the things you're now responsible for as the CEO of your own company, I wonder if you'd even apply for your own job. (I don't think many would – especially not at the pay that is being advertised.)

MY STORY: HOW I LEARNED THESE LESSONS

How do I know this story so well? It's because I've lived it. I started my private practice after I quit my job as a physical therapist in professional soccer at the age of 26. I had absolutely no clue about how to run a real business. At first, I thought it was all about being a great practitioner. I thought that all I had to do was continue to improve my clinical skills and make sure that my patients got results.

And that worked for the first two years or so.

But the inevitable flatline happened and it one day became obvious that there was very little growth in my revenue, despite the time and effort I put into learning new clinical skills.

After being stuck at the same revenue level for a while, I realized that it was time to learn more about this thing called "marketing." I was convinced at this point that my business success was going to be *all* down to how well I could market. So, I went off and learned how to create a marketing system. And it worked. I got inundated with lots more people interested in my services.

But then I realized that getting good at marketing just gave me a new problem –not knowing how to sell my cash-pay services.

My private practice is in the UK – where medicine is completely free to patients, paid for by the government as a form of socialized medicine. There's no co-pay or deductibles. It is just free. It meant I had all these people interested in my service which they assumed would be paid for by the government. As you can imagine, the objections to paying in cash, for what they believed they could get for free, came thick and fast. It exposed that I had no clue how to sell the value of what I do to them. So, I set about learning how to sell effectively at higher prices.

I got pretty good at it and things were okay for a while.

Now at this point, I am a few years into starting my practice and I think I've cracked it. I'm now a great therapist, I'm a good marketer, and I know how to sell. I'm thinking "show me the money."

But all that did was put me in a position where I needed to hire other people to keep up with the demand that my marketing and sales skills created.

And this is where it started to go *really* wrong.

Although I was busier than ever, I was taking home less money than ever. I was doing more but making less. At one point I had more than twenty people on my payroll, all spread across four clinics that were miles apart from each other. I thought what I had was a private practice. What I really had was a hot mess that was a disaster waiting to happen.

The reality of my situation was this: I was a great clinician with skills in marketing and sales – and that just compounded the problem that I didn't really know how to run a real business.

HOW DID I BECOME A BETTER LEADER?

Accepting this, I set off on a new journey to learn yet *another* new business skill. The one that I was looking to learn this time was leadership.

How do I become a better leader? That was the question I asked myself over and over. I assumed that once I found the answer, I could get back to growing and scaling a more profitable practice that I could enjoy owning; one that compensated me fairly for the blood, sweat and tears I was investing.

The problem was this: I fell into the trap that many business owners do when they consider the idea of leadership – thinking that all of my problems would disappear when I became a "better leader." I thought that becoming a "better leader" was the missing piece in the jigsaw, and that once I finished the puzzle, I could sail off into the sunset, sit on the beach somewhere in Florida, and let my employees bring in the cash while I topped up my tan and they topped up my bank account.

If only.

Being a "better leader" is important, but it's certainly not the final piece of the puzzle if you're looking for long-lasting *business* success. Being a good leader only gets you so far before you realize there's a difference between leadership skills and the specific responsibilities and tasks required of a CEO who can lead.

As I've since found out, it's the latter that you need to focus on if you're wanting to be successful in private practice for the long term. There is a huge difference between being a leader and a leader who runs a business. That difference is what we're going to discuss within the pages of this book.

A BETTER LEADER, OR A BETTER CEO?

If, having spent years being a great clinician, you now find yourself in the situation of needing to be a better leader for your business, you are not alone. It is the top job and yet many who occupy it do so by default – not because of merit.

Accepting that you need to become a better leader is the first step toward building a practice that you can be proud to call your own. It is the first step toward owning and running a company that doesn't rely upon you being there every day. It is also the first step to understanding that in order to get a handle on the company you've created, and all of its moving parts, you must become world class at the other role you'll need to play – you, the CEO (Part 2 of this book).

"Leadership" and "business leadership" are two very different things and they come with completely different sets of skills and requirements to be great at either or both.

I believe the question you should ask is not, "How do I become a better leader?" It is, "How do I become a better leader *and* CEO of my clinic?" You should also ask, "What are the specific roles and responsibilities that are required of each?"

When you know the answers to those two questions, your chances of success in private practice are suddenly looking rosier. And that is why I am so glad you've picked up this book. We're going to be answering both of those questions, and a whole lot more.

Having worked closely with many, I've noticed that one of the biggest flaws of many private practice owners is that they never consider themselves to be the CEO of their own companies.

Sure, they think of themselves as business owners – but never as the CEO. That is because most do not know what the CEO's job description actually is, let alone how to be successful in the role.

I know I didn't.

Leadership is a very confusing topic, and any study of it can often leave you feeling like you have to become someone you're not or behave in a way that isn't true to who you are.

Anyone who struggles with leadership privately thinks that it is because they are not born with the "natural" qualities they believe to be required of leaders. They think that because they are unable to inspire and motivate others, or because they can't thump their chests or raise their voices and command people to do things for them, that they are not going to be great leaders. But honestly, none of that is needed. None of that is required for success as a leader in private practice.

Leadership is a construct. It is something that is open for interpretation depending upon the situation that you're in (as a business owner, parent, teacher, etc.).

I believe you can be a great leader in any situation.

That could be as a parent, or a teacher, or just to a group of friends who are looking for someone to lean on or take the lead. Being a leader is a way of living. It is a cap you wear 24/7.

For example, I am a leader when I am at home and with my family. I can choose to live the role of a leader 24/7 and in almost any scenario that you can imagine. However, when I am on the couch with my kids watching Disney, my CEO cap is hanging up at work. *As a CEO, I am doing specific things. As a leader, I am living a certain way.*

If leadership is a construct open to each individual's interpretation, then the role of a CEO is the complete opposite. It involves a specific set of non-negotiable tasks and responsibilities that must be carried out successfully or the company will fail.

These include things like creating a strategic growth plan, setting the annual budget, managing money, creating the marketing strategy, hiring A players, retaining A players, understanding key metrics, coaching people, and developing the company culture (all to be covered in the pages of this book).

This explains why some people are great leaders, but cannot run great companies. I've even spoken to many employees who tell me that their boss is a "great leader" and "very inspiring," and yet their companies continue to fail. It is because the role of the CEO is not being performed correctly.

I think it is very possible to be a great leader – but not necessarily a great CEO. However, I do not believe that it is possible to be a great CEO if you're not a great leader.

Put another way: **the role of CEO comes with a highly specific job description that is easier to execute if you are a great leader.**

SO, WHAT IS LEADERSHIP?

The answer is: it depends. It varies upon the context in which you're using the term. There's a *general* view of leadership that covers all situations you might find yourself in throughout life. Then there is the more specific role of a business leader.

It's very easy for people to think that leadership is a trait or a skill that you're either born with, or not. That you either have the right "personality" for it, or not. That you're ruled out of it if you're an introvert and "in" if you happen to have a powerful presence that is comparable to that of an inspiring politician or great football coach.

We've all seen this stereotype in the movies or on TV. But here's the thing: for every great politician, football coach, or business owner that you can think of who has a strong and charismatic personality, there are tens of thousands of great leaders who are not so charismatic. There are many leaders who are not so loud or vocal in their day-to-day practice, and yet they are at the helm of very successful companies or teams. You don't hear from them because they're introverted, or they just don't like being in the spotlight.

It doesn't mean they're not there – you just don't see them as they're busy running their companies.

Thus, we can conclude early that the secret to being a successful leader doesn't have as much to do with your personality or the tone of your voice as you might currently think. And that should be good news for you. It means there *are* things in your control that determine how good of a leader you will become of your private practice.

Most people think of leadership in the context of *who* you are, and the personality traits you're born with. But I have a much simpler version of what leadership is that has served me very well. Here are the two things that I believe summarize precisely what great leadership is about as it pertains to general situations in life.

1. **Great leaders are able to raise the performance of their people beyond that which they are capable of on their own.**

2. **Great leaders bring certainty to uncertain situations.**

Let's look at both of those points in more detail.

1. **Great leaders are able to raise the performance of their people beyond that which they are capable of on their own.**

What does this mean? However you look at it, this is evident in every scenario in which a great leader exists. Take a football team, for example. For three seasons, the team has underperformed under one coach. The coach is sacked, and a different coach comes in to lead the same group of players. Somehow the new coach is able to lift the team from the bottom of the division to the top tier in a matter of months. It is because the coach – the leader – knows how to get the extra 20 percent in performance from his players. The previous coach hadn't figured that out.

I spent five seasons working in professional soccer and I witnessed this very thing happen twice. After one manager was fired because of a failing team, the new one came in and got more from the same team simply by changing the way he would speak to them. He worked out ways to get them to give him more.

Another scenario is at school. How do some teachers get more from kids when other teachers struggle to get anything? There's always that scenario where that one teacher somehow got more from you than you ever knew was possible. You excelled at English, yet you struggled with history. Two different teachers, two different results. That is leadership in play.

You'll see it at home, too.

On their own, kids can achieve a lot. But with a parent who has a strong leadership presence, kids will obviously go on to achieve so much more.

What about athletes? How do they achieve what they do? They don't do it on their own, that's for sure. No one ever achieves a gold medal without a coach. The coach is also a leader. They're helping those athletes get more from themselves than they ever could on their own. You could go all the way to kids' soccer or Little League. There's a leader there who is coaching the kids to get more from themselves than they could on their own.

Everywhere you look in life, anytime you see someone doing well or excelling, there's a strong leadership influence somewhere in the background, helping that person get more from themselves than they ever could on their own.

Here's another example. I've experienced many instances where other business owners have looked at my staff and wondered how they can land the type of people who work for me.

They look at my team and think that all of their problems would go away if only they could get one or two of my people on their team.

I know they think this way because they tell me to my face.

And when they do, I tell them that they're not thinking accurately. I remind them what they're thinking pre-supposes that my employees would perform the same way for them as they do for me. Because it is very unlikely they will.

How my employees perform for me is the *effect* – the cause is *how they are led*.

If I am great at leadership, it is because I have great people. And equally, if I have a great team, it is because of great leadership.

It is a mutually beneficial relationship that cannot be broken by either side. It means that you can poach my staff – but you are unlikely to get what my staff currently give me unless you are willing to do what I do.

2. Great leaders bring certainty to uncertain situations.

As I wrote this book, the COVID-19 pandemic had just begun. It is inarguably the biggest medical and economic crisis to hit the planet in the last 100 years, and the reality is that no one knows for sure how to deal with the uncertainty that it is bringing.

It's a potent cocktail of a global health emergency and a financial catastrophe sprinkled with a lot of fake news and polarizing politicized opinions. It has created a level of uncertainty that was previously unseen or even dreamt of.

During this time, people are looking for leadership. They're desperate for it. Millions of people are tuning in to the daily updates from their president or prime minister, hoping to find some certainty to help them feel better about the situation. This is the job of leadership. To make people feel better about things they think are out of their control.

Being effective at leadership requires the management of one's own emotions when all the people around you are looking for help with their own.

The world might be falling down around you, but you can't let anyone see that you're affected by it. You might be having some trouble in your personal life, but you can't let it shake you. You might have had your clinic closed down by the government (enforced by a lockdown) and all of your revenue streams cut off, but you can't let that alter how you speak to and present yourself to your employees.

Put another way, if you can't manage your own emotions, you can't manage someone else's. It is that simple.

Good leaders are confident in themselves and they know that the best and only way to help the people around them is through certainty in their own actions and behaviors. Far from worrying over what others think about how or what they're doing, good leaders are certain that what they're doing (and how they're doing it) brings a much-needed level of calmness and direction to the situation.

I've learned that the best leaders are not always right – they don't need to be. They just need to be certain in their own heads that they are.

But if they find out later that they weren't, they're humble enough – and certain enough – to admit it.

Great leaders are certain even when they don't know all the answers. They won't hide from the fact that they don't know something or can't yet see a way through. But the way they admit to *not knowing* is the part that makes them great leaders. They're confident about the fact that they don't know. They're able to look people in the eye and stand tall as they announce they have "no clue" what the right answer is, but that they'll figure it out.

I think this is one of the best characteristics of a great leader. Leadership is not knowing everything, it is being comfortable with acknowledging that you don't know everything and committing to resolving the situation regardless.

Yet, that's the complete opposite direction that most people seem to be headed in today's society.

Too many people are trying to fake knowing everything out of fear that they'll be judged by others if they don't.

It's creating a society where people feel constantly inferior – yet project an outward view of looking superior. It creates mental and emotional turmoil for that person, not to mention pent up anger and resentment.

It's a recipe for disaster for anyone who is aiming to achieve anything of significance in their life – such as feeling in control of it.

I believe it's better to publicly admit you don't know something and privately commit to resolving it. After all, you're always rewarded in public for the work you do in private.

You could very easily apply this idea to an interaction you have with a patient. If they ask you how long it will take to fix their hamstring injury and you stumble and stall over your answer, or you immediately break eye contact with them or change the tone of your voice (because you're not certain), you've just lost their trust.

You're still their physical therapist, but you're no longer a leader in their eyes.

What they need and want (just as much as your great clinical skills) is to be in the care of a great leader, someone who is certain in himself. After all, if you're not certain in yourself how can they be certain you can do what they need?

"I HAVE ABSOLUTELY NO CLUE WHAT IS COMING NEXT"

And it's the same with your staff – they need to know that you aren't faking it or pandering to their needs. I can vividly recall an interview that I did with the lady who heads the operations of my now-global media business. At the end of the interview, she asked me the standard question that goes something like, "What are the career progression opportunities for this role?"

After she asked me, I sat back in my chair and went silent for a few seconds while I looked out of the window. I came back with the following reply:

"You know, I have absolutely no clue what the opportunities will be. All I know is that this company is going as fast as a rocket ship en-route to the moon and more good things are happening than I ever thought possible. For me to sit here and tell you what might or might not happen – just to appease you, because that is what I am supposed to do right now – would be me blowing smoke up your ass. The truth is I have absolutely no clue what will happen, but I know it is going to be fun getting to where we are going. If you want to jump on board, I'll make sure you know about opportunities as they open up."

Cue the startled look on her face.

We got our relationship off to a great start because she immediately knew who she was working for – someone who is certain even when he doesn't know the answer; someone who wouldn't pander or lie about things. Even if I didn't know the answers to her future questions, she'd get the truth. Without attempting to blow smoke up my own ass, I believe that is a sign of great leadership.

Okay, so that's the end of the first chapter. What I want you to take from it is the idea that leadership in life and leadership in business are two very different things requiring very different skills and attributes. To be successful in private practice you're going to have to excel in both. As we move through the rest of this book together, my aim is to shed light on the difference and help you understand what is required of you, the leader and you, the CEO of a private practice. I'll explain the personal qualities that I believe great leaders have and we'll also pay a lot of attention to the important roles and tasks that should capture every CEO's focus.

In fact, we'll work through the actual job description of a CEO (you'll need to download your copy: **www.paulgough.com/leadership-resource**) so that you're crystal clear on what you should be doing and how to get better at your role.

It's going to be very enlightening for you.

Come with me to the next chapter. We'll start by clearing up the answer to that age-old question everyone in business has: "What is the difference between a manager and a leader?" Turn the page to find out!

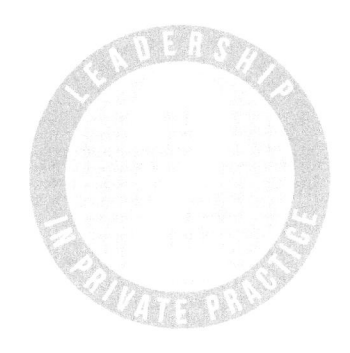

WHAT'S THE DIFFERENCE BETWEEN A MANAGER AND LEADER?

If the difference between a leader and a CEO is misunderstood, then the difference between a manager and a leader is even more so. It is yet another thing in business ownership that is not clearly defined and, as such, it leaves people confused about what role to play and when.

Could it be possible that you play both roles as a private practice owner? I believe so. In fact, I believe that *leadership evolves as a result of management excellence.*

What is more, the two are interwoven.

In the beginning, as you start your company, you are the manager *and* leader – of yourself. Then, as you bring on your first employees, you begin to manage and lead other people. From there, your leadership role evolves. You're managing and leading simultaneously, but you just might not acknowledge or recognize it. You're telling people what to do to make sure the business is operationally efficient (manager) and, at the same time, you're getting the best out of them (leader). You're also bringing a sense of certainty to them when the business experiences early challenges or setbacks (leader).

Personally, I don't think it matters too much what you call yourself or how you self-identify. What matters most is your understanding of the fact that you do have to play both roles – and there's a clear difference in what is required of each role if you want to be successful.

I think much of the confusion that surrounds the difference between manager and leader comes from our own egos. It is much more exciting to say that you're a leader as opposed to a manager.

As proof, look at the number of books written and sold on the topic of leadership versus those written about management. What is more, leaders are often glamorized as strong, passionate, and charismatic types who make big things happen and everyone feel great. At least, that is what the Hollywood movies want you to believe. This means every business owner wants to think of herself as the leader – but in comparison, very few people want to think of themselves as a manager.

And let's be honest, manager even *sounds* like harder work, doesn't it?

If you're confused, just think about it like this:

"We are all managers who need to know how to lead."

Another way to think of it is this:

"Your title is 'manager' – but your people make you a leader."

No matter how big your company gets, you're always going to have to play both roles. Even if you employ 400 people, you're not exempt from managing. Because of the way the company organizational chart works, you still have dozens of people reporting directly to you. You will always be both managing and leading.

If leading is about setting the vision, then being a manager is about ensuring that the necessary standards are met to achieve that vision. Standards usually disappear when the leader is thinking about growth. It's why it's so important that both roles are evident in your practice.

The owner of a practice can do both of these things. The operational or general manager of the practice can do both as well – it is just more common that the owner is the one responsible for coming up with the vision or the specific outcomes for the practice.

I think it is vital that you – the private practice owner – are happy to do both of these things, particularly in the early or rapid-growth years (the first five years or so).

And at the same time, do not get too hung up on the fact that the people around you are not the leader that you are. You don't need them to be. You just need them to lead at a level above the people they are directly responsible for managing on the company org chart (I've included a copy of an example org. chart in the toolkit that accompanies this book: **www.paulgough.com/leadership-resource**).

And that, in essence, is how a company leadership team is developed.

When you have a head of marketing, a head of sales, a head of operations, and a head of finance, you have what is commonly called a *leadership team*.

They may not be *the* leaders of the company, but they are able to act and think like leaders at a level above anyone else in the company. In that way, they are leading. But they also still need to be managed – and led – by you.

TRAFFIC POLICE VS. COACH

Here's an easy way to think about the differences between each role. Managers act a lot like traffic police, and leaders act like football coaches. Figuratively speaking, managers are responsible for making sure that the traffic is flowing in the right direction and at the right speed – and that no one is crashing into each other.

In this way, the manager ensures things keep running smoothly. Essentially, they're making sure the growth plan that the business owner created is being executed correctly (more on that later). They're ensuring that people are doing their jobs and processes are being followed. They're telling people when to slow down and when to go faster, depending upon the results being generated.

That doesn't mean that the owner of the business can't and shouldn't get involved this type of work. When needed, you should. But you shouldn't be spending *all* of your time in what I call the "nitty gritty" or the "tactical stuff" that is often the job of the people farther down the org chart.

You have to develop the skill to know when you need to float between the two types of work, as and when your business needs.

And that need is constantly changing.

For example, in the beginning, when you started your clinic, it was likely that you had lots of grand visions for the future of the company. One minute you're thinking about how many clinics you would like to own and what it would be like to one day sell your chain of 25 clinics for $20 million. Then, just a few seconds later, you're back into the day-to-day of the practice, having to update the process for billing an insurance company or dealing with a patient on the phone who wants to cancel their appointment.

The latter are examples of the nitty gritty, tactical things – the weeds – that are very important for a business to manage correctly if it is to run smoothly.

However, the business owner that spends all of his time doing these things soon finds himself stuck. Crises require tactics. Sustained success requires strategy. If you're always in a crisis, is it because you're always working tactically?

If you're spending all of your time on the tactical things that are often below your pay grade, you'll find you're always paid at a grade less than you hoped.

Whether you like your business or not, it does not discriminate against you. Your business always pays out at the level at which you work. If you do $15 per hour work, that is what you get paid. If you do $500 per hour work, in the end, that is what you get paid. In the long run, it is fair. It doesn't always seem that way to business owners, but that is mostly because of how they choose to spend the most valuable asset available to a business owner – time.

Here's something very important for you to grasp: your business can only ever grow when you're thinking strategically and considering what it needs to be able to grow, not just operate.

There's a big difference between doing work that merely delivers on promises already made – and that which drives the company forward. The work you need to do to grow hasn't happened yet. It's in the future – it's waiting to be created. Its value has yet to be realized and it doesn't happen when you're thinking tactically about things like social media, another new website, or what questions to ask to stop a patient from objecting to your prices.

Business growth work requires you to be thinking about your company structure, developing your people, getting a better return on your marketing investment, or improving the sales process so that you can scale.

Business growth is a direct result of the type of work that the owner chooses to do. If it is all tactical – nitty gritty – then the business will stay at its current level. It's why the leader must think strategically as much as possible. It's why your day and your week must be optimized in the best way possible to allow you to do more of this strategic thinking.

And sure, there *could* be more growth if you work harder on the tactics. But it usually comes at a price – that being your health or not seeing your kids.

No matter what anyone else tells you, you cannot work ten times harder and expect to make ten times more money. Society has you believing that "working harder" is the secret to making money. But I assure you, it is not true. It really isn't about how hard you work. It's about the type of work you choose to do and how much of it you do.

The ability to allocate time and the prioritization of the activities you choose to work on are the ultimate skills required of a CEO. It is what defines how successful you are in life and in business. We all have the same time available to us – what we choose to do with it determines the success we get.

Of course, it also means there's another side to this equation.

If you're guilty of doing too much tactical work and getting stuck there, you can also be guilty of doing too much of the "visionary" stuff, too.

Any business owner who is spending all day dreaming of how the business will *one day* look – but is not willing to be on the ground floor to do the things needed bring the vision to life – inevitably finds that the vision becomes a nightmare he can't escape. The key is to be able to be great at both – just learn when and for how long you need to do either.

BEHIND EVERY GREAT LEADER IS A "DOER"

If business leaders need to be more strategic in their thinking, then managers need to be great "doers." A "doer" ensures the business owner's big vision comes to life. If the leader is spending 80 percent of her time thinking strategically about the growth plan, the manager is spending 80 percent of his time making sure milestones are being hit to ensure growth occurs.

Basically, "doers" are vital to the success of your company and you must have one around you.

What you often find, though, is the founder of the company wears the name badge of leader – but gets stuck at the level of perpetually "doing." A business that has been stuck at the same level for some time is a classic symptom of a leader who is guilty of *too much doing* and not enough strategic thinking.

(Can you relate?)

Worse, they can often find that they've actually hired someone to "do stuff" – but are still doing it themselves. This business owner is definitely overworked and getting very little in the way of rewards for it. They are the leader in name, but not in how they think or act.

Another classic symptom of a business owner who is stuck at the level of constantly "doing" is that they operate and make decisions from a place of pent-up emotion. They are constantly "shooting from the hip" or "flying off the handle" when faced with even the smallest of setbacks.

If there's a screwup at the front desk causing a billing issue, or yet another mix up with a patient scheduling at the wrong time, it's easy to keep venting at the people involved, yelling at them to follow the process you created.

You can keep shouting and keep yelling. But what if the person you're shouting at simply isn't capable of following the process? What good is yelling or, for that matter, even fixing the process?

The solution to the pain point is only found when you find the real problem causing it. In this case, it is likely the recruitment, onboarding, and training process in the company that needs fixing. There is a *design* change in the business operating system that needs to be made to fix the issue at the source. However, if you're stuck working tactically, you can't see this and so you keep firing from the hip and keep flying off the handle every time something happens. At some point, you have to realize that a different approach is needed – one that is strategic.

HOW YOU RUN YOUR LIFE IS HOW YOU RUN YOUR BUSINESS

If any of that sounds familiar, and you find yourself constantly fighting fires or always feeling like you're "spinning your wheels," always fixing the same problems over and over again, then it's possible you need to spend more time thinking about the structure and design of your business than working in it.

After all, structure brings freedom.

Function follows form.

And, by the way, it is the same in life!

If you want a terrific life, you've got to design it before you live it. You've got to think about the conditions, standards, and values of your life as much as the rewards you want from it.

Designing your life and living it really are two very different things. And personally, I think this is where so many people go wrong in pursuit of happiness or fulfillment.

There's no shortage of people who want to "live their best life," but there is a huge shortage of people who are prepared to design it first in order to make living it a reality. I don't see many T-shirts with the slogan "Design Your Life First" on the front. But I do see T-shirts with something like the words "One Life, Live It," insinuating that all you have to do is show up every day and play.

Sadly, that isn't how it works in life or in business.

If you look at most people, they really *do* want to live a great life – there's no shortage of desire. But sadly, they're not doing that (at least not at the level they want).

And it's the same with business owners.

They really do want a great business. No one starts a business and wants it to be crappy. But years later, and despite a lot of effort and sacrifice, they still don't have a successful one. There's no shortage of determination or hard work. The will is there, but they are lacking the direction. And it nearly always happens because they lack the strategic oversight to achieve it. That is a business skill that can be learned.

Over the years, I've discovered that there's not that much difference between business success and life success. That is because both have one thing in common: the person living it or owning it.

One of my favorite sayings is "How you run your life is how you run your business." It basically means the same behaviors and level of thinking show up at home or in the office. The equivalent good and bad habits appear in both areas.

Said differently, there's no running to a phone booth to become Superman just before your business opens its doors. You are Clark Kent at home *and* in the practice.

I believe the primary reason that people don't have the life they want is because they spend too much time thinking about the things and stuff they think they *need* in their life for it to be great.

Instead of thinking about *how* to actually achieve them, thoughts are consumed by ownership of things like cars, TVs, glamorous vacations, or big houses.

It's the same for business owners – they obsess over wanting more patients and more money rather than what is required to do so: the how, the strategy.

And, what is more, because their thoughts are relentlessly fixed on "getting more" (both money and patients), there are very few, if any, thoughts about if either will actually make you happy. Many presuppose they automatically will.

But I am not sure that they always do.

Getting patients and making money is one thing – but if you're not careful, it can come at the expense of finding happiness and fulfillment in your life. And surely that is what you want from your business? I believe a business is simply a vehicle for a terrific life and I build my life around my business to suit.

My Uncle Liam always used to say to me, "Paul, making money is easy – it is the other stuff in life that is difficult." Back then I never believed him. I looked at a lot of people around me who didn't have money and assumed it must be difficult to make a lot of it. But if the truth be told,

I really didn't know what he meant by "the other stuff." Now I get it. He was talking about living and getting the best from your life every day.

After all, you can sit in an Uber for twenty hours per day, 365 days per year, and you'll make a decent sum of money. Certainly enough to get by. But is it going to give you the fulfillment and contentment you want in life?

Maybe. But probably not.

Therefore, it surely has to be about *how* you make your money – not just how much you make. That is why the strategy, or the design aspect of your business (and life), is so important.

What is the point in having made a load of money if you've never seen your son play baseball or you've never been able to pick him up from school because you were always looking for more patients and more money? It is the strategy that dictates how the money is made and ultimately if the juice is worth the squeeze.

Bottom line, the right strategies for your life and business are vital. These strategies require time to be invested, not to mention skills honed, if you're going to become world class.

CHOICE DICTATES QUALITY OF LIFE

I believe that what we're all after as business owners is the freedom of choice. Not freedom, but the freedom to choose. There's a difference. If you're lucky enough to live in the western world, you're already free. But you might not feel it. And that's because there's a lack of freedom of choice.

People tell me they want to be free from their practice – but I think what they're *really* saying is they want to be free to choose when they can be at or away from it. They don't want to feel like they're shackled to it 365 days per year. They want the choice to come and go when it suits them, go on vacation when they want, and be home for dinner or soccer any night they wish.

Remember this: *the people with the best lives have the best choices*. You don't want more options – it's more important to have choices. Everyone has options. Options are all around us – but not everyone has choices.

Choices are things you can actually execute on. Options are things that are available to everyone and in the western world there's no shortage of options for things you could do or get. But for most people, there is a serious lack of actual choice that can become a reality.

For example, everyone has the *option* to book a first-class seat on an airline – but not everyone has the means to actually *choose* to book one. And everyone has the *option* to live in a big house with a swimming pool out back – but not everyone can actually *choose* to do so as they don't have the means.

Every day I wake up, I do so with the intention of expanding the number of choices available to me. Remember this: the quality of your life is directly proportional to the number of choices available in your life. Increasing life choices is the number one objective for me and why I am in business in the first place.

If you focus on more money, you might just find that you get it, but you've now got more restrictions and liabilities therefore you can't do anything with it. So, what was the point?

If you focus on choice, you can still achieve the money but the decisions you make along the way come with careful consideration of how or if what you're about to do is going to expand your life choices – or limit them.

Focusing on more money is great. But be careful what you wish for. You might just get all the money you want but find that you're more restricted than ever and no happier for having it.

Try it for yourself. Switch your focus to being about expanding the number of life choices available to you and your family. I promise you, the quality of your life and the fulfillment you get will increase exponentially. What is more, you'll likely find your desire to buy things or get stuff that you once thought you needed to be happy decreases.

I've learned that when you have the choice, you realize that is all you ever wanted in the first place. Actually, getting the thing you thought you wanted or needed rarely makes you happy in the long term. Focusing on expanding your choices brings a new level of quality to your life that means you're not working on *getting* more things. Rather, you're focused on *achieving* more things.

It's hard to explain, but it's a wonderful place to get to in life.

Give it a try and come and join me.

MAKE YOUR LIFE ABOUT ACCOMPLISHMENT – NOT ACTIVITY

I would encourage anyone who is serious about getting more from their life to think about the design aspect of life – the structure. It includes how your day will look, what time you want available for yourself, who you want to work with, what standards you'll accept from others around you, what level of discipline you need, and the areas in which you need it. Doing this will take you well above the need for more things and stuff.

At this level, you're no longer focused on just making it through the day or hustling for more dollars. No, you're focused on the longer term and higher outcome of your life. You're at a much higher level in your life.

Getting to a higher level in your thinking elevates you above the noise that is likely to be consuming your day. Getting above the noise allows you to see who is doing all of the shouting in the first place. And that's a vital thing for a business owner to be able to do. If you can't see the forest for the trees, you don't know what is waiting in there for you.

As a business owner, you have to be able to see past the trees so that you can see what is coming down the line in terms of problems and opportunities. If you're constantly engulfed in the same problems – in life or business – and there's very little if any progress, it's likely because you're living and thinking day to day.

Get your head up high. Instead of a relentless "doer," become an observer of the things happening around you. Do not constantly react to each one.

One of the best things I learned through the early phases of the coronavirus pandemic was to become an observer of the things that were happening to me.

I resisted the temptation to have strong opinions or form judgements about things that people were doing or saying around me. I began to realize that when I step back from constantly being engulfed in the situation – having thoughts about it or wanting to express my opinion on it – I was becoming less affected by the events that were literally bringing the world to its knees. I began to apply that same methodology to running my business and it's helped tremendously.

If you can learn to see beyond the end of the day or past the current drama and think well beyond next week or even next month, you can picture your end goal. You can start to see the top of the mountain that you're climbing as you build your business. This allows you to start thinking about how you want your life and business to look in the next three to five years from now – and when you see it, work backward.

I always say that if I can see it – or I can see someone else doing it – then I can make it happen. I just need to be able to see it. And once you can see what you really want, you can start to build a roadmap that shows you how to achieve it. This allows you to think about all of the things you will need to do, as well as the likely challenges that will hit you along the way to getting wherever it is you want to go.

The best thing about living this way – in both life and business – is that when the inevitable challenges come along, they don't affect you nearly as much as others who are experiencing the same setback.

Why?

Simply because you were expecting them. And because you were, you dealt with them better than the next person.

I always say, "The problem is never the problem." The only *real* problem in life is that we weren't expecting a problem. And because we weren't expecting it, what follows from this is often a poor response to the unexpected problem. And that nearly always creates an even worse situation. *That's* what hurts you – how badly you responded, or the bad decision you made to fix it. But it's rarely, if ever, the issue itself.

If I get hit and I was expecting it, I likely have a plan to get back up faster than the person who didn't expect it. It's that simple. If you can see things coming, you get to dodge the bullets, or they start skimming off you. Doing just this – in both business and life – immediately puts you ahead of most people.

The key, though, and where it all starts, is getting yourself out of the day-to-day grind, putting your workaholic ego aside and spending more time *thinking* about what you really want and *how* you're going to get it.

Then, of course, executing on it. Get busy hustling only once you've got your roadmap. But don't hustle for hustling's sake. That's dumb. And the only thing you're going to get is tired.

Thinking – *real thinking*, where you are actually considering ideas and concepts that are not immediately obvious to you – is a grossly underestimated sport. Yet, for those who play it regularly, the prize is huge. It leads to less frustration, less hassle, less stress – and, dare I say it, even less work (the "doing work," that is).

Make your life about accomplishment – not activity. You can't take activity to the bank and cash it. Don't let your life become about moving in favor of momentum. There is a huge difference between the two.

Don't focus on the instant gratification that comes with getting stuff done, either. Instead, become more strategic and critical in your thinking – and start asking yourself if what you got done today was "growth work" or "grunt work." When you think critically, you can see eleven other solutions to the problems that no one else can.

Stop telling your staff to do the same thing every time they ask you the same question. Instead, spend time on designing a more effective training manual that they can reference whenever needed so they don't have to ask you ever again.

Stop constantly blaming and changing marketing when you have poor leads. Instead, focus on recruitment and training the people who answer your phone so they are able to turn "okay" leads into high-paying patients.

Don't focus on getting a long-overdue bill from an insurance company finally paid and being happy that you did. Instead, focus on finding out why the delay keeps happening in the first place and what part of the company needs to be redesigned to ensure it never happens again.

Don't keep wasting time on hiring and firing dummies, constantly blaming the job market in your area. Instead, design a better recruitment process that finds and picks out A players (more on that in a later chapter).

These are all examples of where you, as a private practice owner, could change the level of your thinking and as a result change your outcome.

Remember this: you can't solve a problem with the level of thinking that got you into it. *Tactical thinking* creates constant problems requiring a lot of effort with very little forward momentum. *Strategic thinking* creates breakthroughs and solutions that take you to a level of living that you currently can't begin to imagine.

Strategic thinking is the only way to achieve long-lasting success in business. And to get breakthroughs in your thinking, to get the strategic idea, you need to allocate a significant amount of time to it. The quality of your thinking is directly proportional to the amount of time you allocate to it.

Put another way, you need to spend more than the customary five minutes doing it. Everything that you think about in the first five to ten minutes of your thinking session is something you already knew. It was likely what you had already considered to solve your problem. The breakthroughs – the solutions – are usually found twenty, thirty, forty minutes or longer into your session. The question is, will you as the leader of your company afford yourself the time to do it?

GET YOUR FREE RESOURCE KIT: PAULGOUGH.COM/LEADERSHIP-RESOURCE

As this chapter comes to an end, I want you to take away these two points:

1. There's a difference between being a manager and a leader, but you'll always need to do both as the owner of a business. The most important thing is to recognize how much time you're spending on both. The beginning and early years of your business are a constant wrestling match played out between leading and managing. As you get more staff and a leadership team around you, it's about spending 80 percent of your time on the strategic thinking that allows your company to find new paths to grow. If you're not great at doing stuff, it's vital you employ someone who is so that you can focus on the bigger-picture stuff.

2. You are only as good as your level of thinking and the time you allocate to it. If you want a better business – and a better life – then spend more time thinking about the design and structure of your life and *how* you will get it (not just getting it). Time is your greatest asset. How you invest it – or spend it – is up to you.

I've touched on the idea of people a few times in this chapter, and how they can assist your or hold you back in pursuit of your business goals. Come with me to the next chapter and we'll talk more about how to get the best from your people.

IT'S ALL ABOUT THE PEOPLE

When you start your business, it is all about the customer. Yet, for it to keep growing, it has to become about the people – your staff. Put another way, when and if your business reaches a flatline, it's probably because you're still focused on getting more patients and providing better service to patients – as opposed to finding and growing the right people to serve those patients for you. The difference is profound.

As a leader, you are only as good as your people. People are the foundation of any great company's success. Every ounce of value that your clients receive has its roots in your people. It's not the number of your qualifications that make the difference – it's the quality of your people. It means one of the primary tasks you have as a leader is to hire well and help people be successful in their roles (and lives).

You need them to be successful at delivering value, and you as the leader have a big hand to play in making that happen.

You can't just employ people and expect them to do it. That isn't how it works. You have to create the environment and set standards that allow them to grow and develop during their time with you so that they're able to feel successful in their position.

Does leading people come with frustrations? Of course. Does it come with inconsistencies and unpredictability? You bet it does. But it *can* be very exciting and hugely rewarding to watch your people grow.

I've said many times that this is one of the things I enjoy most about being a business owner. I get the opportunity to watch people come into my world and grow into someone they didn't know they were capable of becoming. And when they come into my world, I care more about how they develop as *people* than employees. I am not so much watching how they are as employees as I am how they are as *people*.

That is because the telephone script takes care of itself if they have the confidence to follow it. The customer service protocol is easy to follow if they have the confidence to greet patients with a smile and a hug. The treatment takes care of itself if they are comfortable with being vulnerable enough to open up about their own personal life stories with patients many years older than themselves.

I've had some staff work with me for more than ten years and in that time I've watched young girls become strong, confident women. I've watched them get married and have kids and go on to become amazing parents. I've had staff come to me with huge confidence issues when they first started. Months later, they felt more comfortable and happier because of their working environment and the other people they're paired with.

WATCH OUT FOR "TWIN B" ARRIVING AT WORK

I've employed countless people and one thing I can tell you is that the ones who are progressing in their personal lives are the ones progressing in their work lives. It is rarely the other way around. Issues with a partner at home can easily derail their focus or productivity at work. Yet, doing well at work rarely solves a bad marriage.

Think about all of the employees you've ever had.

I bet you will see a pattern: the ones who *stop* developing their work ethic, their habits, and their standards are the ones who often are your most difficult-to-manage employees. They become the alter ego you didn't see in the interview.

They become what I call "Twin B." Their success in your role will be defined by how well Twin B performs.

"Twin A" is the one who interviews well – but "Twin B" is the one who eventually shows up for the job. Sadly, "Twin B" is the worse version and is the one that causes you the problems.

"Twin A" interviewed great – he was a great actor. "Twin B" shows up about 90 days later and often brings personal issues to work or looks for problems that don't exist. They're bored or lacking attention in their own life, so creating issues or drama at work is their way of adding a little excitement to it. When they start the fire, they get something to moan about to friends or a few likes on Facebook from their friends who are just as sad and miserable.

They'll blame work for their frustrations. Really, work is a scapegoat for the person truly responsible for the roadblocks they've hit in their lives – themself. And, most often, the boredom they're experiencing elsewhere in their lives. Discovering Tinder (the dating app) usually distracts them for a few weeks, but in the end "Twin B" returns. You've got to recognize and get rid of these people ASAP.

I'm not saying that I have had a great relationship with everyone who has ever worked for me. Far from it. There have been many times when people have come to work with me only to leave abruptly because our standards and values were not aligned.

Usually, it was because I recruited incorrectly, or the person was not coachable. Many times – most times – it's that they simply didn't like being held accountable. And that's a huge problem in my companies because accountability is a big part of what I value. They tell me in an interview they love "accountability." It's just that we have different versions of it. I want to hold them accountable, but they seem to think they can do it alone.

The minute they tell me they like to hold themselves accountable, I know we're going in different directions. Why? Because it's not possible to hold yourself accountable for a sustained period of time. It is why all of the top CEOs and sports performers have coaches to hold them to account.

INDEPENDENTLY SUCCESSFUL: THE REAL MEASURE OF SUCCESS

In many ways, being a boss is a lot like being a father. It is an amazing privilege that I never take for granted. As a father, my job is to ensure that my children become independently successful. It is not about helping them be successful when I am around – it is about them being successful whether I am around or not.

As I see it, if they are dependent upon me for the things they want in their lives, then I am not able to call myself a success as a father. I can provide love, a roof over their heads, and food on the table, but those are the entry-level requirements of a father. The ultimate measure of success is to be independently successful without me.

It is the same with your staff – you want to help them to be successful *independent* of you being there. You cannot be there every minute of every day for them to plug into if you seriously expect them to develop.

Even though you might know how to do something better, at some point you have to let your staff figure out how to deal with a challenge on their own. They have to be allowed to do it without your input and you have to be okay even if it doesn't go right. Sometimes the best price to pay is a lesson learned.

Your people give you a significant chunk of their lives. I think it's only fair that we give them back more than just a salary or a health insurance plan. Anyone can do that for them. More than anything, I think the best thing you can do for your people is just *believe in them* more than they believe in themselves.

And that really isn't hard.

Most people have more belief in the tooth fairy or Santa Claus than they do themselves. That's because by the time they've reached adulthood, people have had their belief in their self figuratively knocked out of them.

Being a kid, everything is easy.

Everyone wants to support you and tell you everything is possible, and that you can achieve anything if you wish hard enough. As an adult, the truth hits home that it takes more than just the fact that your mother wants you to achieve things to actually achieve them. Setbacks and disappointments are aplenty. This leads to people perpetually doubting what and even *if* they can achieve anything. Sometimes – many times – they'll bring this self-doubt with them to your work. And that's now your problem to handle. Ignore it at your peril.

GET YOUR FREE RESOURCE KIT: PAULGOUGH.COM/LEADERSHIP-RESOURCE

To really believe in them, you've got to believe they're capable of achieving more than they are now – whatever their circumstance or excuses.

People love to find excuses and give you reasons for their failures, often before they've even taken on a task. I've learned to ignore most of those excuses, simply because it's nearly always just a bad habit they have formed.

As a business owner, you need to recognize the self-limiting beliefs that your people have and encourage them to see past their own doubts. If you don't, it's going to cost you money and limit their personal progress.

REFUSE TO ACCEPT POOR STANDARDS

If you really do want to help them make a change, another way to do it is to refuse to allow them to accept poor standards for themselves.

When and if standards drop in your practice, remind them that they're not letting *you* down, they're letting *themselves* down.

This is a radically different approach that most bosses would never consider taking. Think about it, though. If you think that they're letting you down, you are taking it personally. You think and feel that they're doing it to *you*. You think that because you're paying them, if they don't do something you expected or did something they shouldn't, that they've let *you* down.

But that isn't the way it is.

No way.

The reverse is actually true.

They've let *themselves* down.

You fulfilled your obligation. You set the standards that they agreed to when they took the job. *They* showed up late or *they* didn't do the work required. They've let themselves down in doing so. When you see it this way, it helps both of you.

First, you won't get frustrated, which means you're not going to make a rash, emotional decision or close your mind off from great ideas or opportunities you would otherwise miss for your business.

Second, the only way change *really* occurs is if someone realizes and wants it for himself. I am sure my people want to work for me. They want me to think highly of them. But I know they really want to work for, and have a higher opinion of, themselves.

You want to motivate people and make a real change, but you can't do it for them. Only they can do that. You can provide inspiration, but that doesn't last long. If you want lasting change, you can only change the standards in your company to increase the odds of this happening. When you raise the standards, they often step up – or step out. Either way, you win.

START BY RAISING YOUR OWN STANDARDS

The best place to start is with yourself and raising your own standards. Take it upon yourself to set higher standards in your life and in your work. Wherever those standards are now, you can raise them. Not only will you benefit directly from that personally, but the added benefit is that your people will also be pulled up to a new, higher standard at the same time.

If you're able to set your own standards at a level just above than theirs, and you're showing them a path to get up there with you, then you are pulling them up to higher heights – new heights that they can't, or wouldn't, achieve on their own.

Best, if they can do the same for the people in their lives, you've pulled a lot of others up with you because of the standards you set.

Now you're really inspiring change. And personally, I think this is one of the most rewarding aspects of being a leader.

Don't overlook any of what I am talking about here. A lack of confidence and self-belief is very real. It is what stops most people from ever achieving their full potential. Plus, don't forget that very few people actually have great role models to emulate. You can be that person for them.

Now you're *really* leading.

If you want to make a difference in your practice, don't think it is just achieved by giving people money. Help people believe in themselves more. It is the greatest thing you can do for them. Help them realize that they are the ones who can change their own predicaments. Help people realize that the only person they need to believe in them is the one staring back at them in the mirror. If they do that, the money they want to make will take care of itself.

Helping people to be independently successful is the most important thing you can ever do – whatever your position or title, but definitely if you are a boss.

YOUR PEOPLE NEED THREE SPECIFIC THINGS FROM YOU

If you really want your people to develop and grow into great employees, they're going to need three specific things from you. They are as follows:

1. Support:

Supporting your people means giving them the things they need to be successful. Make sure they've got the best equipment or resources and that they're trained appropriately. Sometimes it is as simple as making sure they've got the time they need to do their job properly. It isn't always about improving their *capability* to do their job – it's often making sure they've got the *capacity* to do it. Are you asking them to do too much and is that the reason they're struggling?

Of course, they also need the right tools and information to give them any chance to be successful in their roles. Support starts with them knowing exactly what it takes to be successful in the role – not "how hard" they have to work, but what result they need to achieve.

Spell it out to them so there can be no mistaking what constitutes success. If you ask most people what their job is, they'll say something binary such as "Answer the phone" or "Treat patients." But that isn't their job – that is something they do on the way to doing their job. Their job is to achieve something specific that is clearly defined – by you.

It could be something like "Ensure patient satisfaction is above eight out of ten" or "Get five additional new patient referrals per week." Once they know specifically what it is, it is much easier to achieve.

Then, when you're both clear on that, you can help them develop the skills needed to achieve it so that they are more likely to want to stay with you for the long-term. Which, as you will find out in a later chapter, is one of the key factors to growing a successful company and keeping your best people in your practice.

Ultimately, support means that you're prepared to continually help them grow and develop the skills that allow them to be successful.

2. Respect:

Everyone on your team is different. As such, they must be treated differently. Whoever said "Everyone must be treated the same" must have been drunk. You treat everyone with the same level of respect as human beings – but you cannot treat everyone the same simply because they're *not all the same*. They each have different career goals and life choices.

You treat them with respect, and you treat them fairly. In doing that, you are then treating them the same, but in the way that they need. It is not a one-size-fits-all model.

Your job as leader is to figure out what they need from you, how they want to be spoken to, and what they value – and then accommodate them in a way that still allows the business to be successful.

The very fact that you're being sensitive to all of their individual needs means you are treating everyone with respect and, above all, you're being fair.

3. Trust:

Trust is the vital ingredient in every relationship. It is the glue that keeps all relationships together. And yet, a lack of it is one of the most common issues in the employee-employer relationship.

If you don't trust your staff to do their jobs, you have a huge problem. You will be tied to the treatment room for the rest of your life and your practice will stop growing. You'll never get a vacation and, even if you do, you will spend the whole seven days paranoid or constantly checking your email for updates. You will be on vacation in body only – your mind will be back at the practice.

It's easy for a business owner to say that they don't trust their staff. As if the problem is all with the employee.

But I think that the real issue here is that the employer simply doesn't trust himself. He doesn't always trust his own recruitment decisions and isn't really clear on the point at which the employee is actually deemed competent, let alone how to get the employee to that point.

I also think a lack of trust exposes huge insecurity problems. The owner often thinks that an employee doing something wrong could spell the end of their business. And if their self-worth is tied to the success of their business, it means that they think they'll be seen as a failure.

I think you need to be really careful about allowing thinking like this to continue. Tying the success of your company to the success of your life is a very dangerous game to play and leads to more pressure being placed on you than you might realize. It is not a healthy place to be, nor does it make for favorable conditions to actually run a successful business.

To get over this, you have to change your view that *you're* a failure if your business fails. But first, and perhaps harder, is that you also have to do the complete opposite: not call yourself a success just because your business is.

Either needs to be irrelevant in the grand scheme of who you are and what your life is about. Business is part of your life. It is a feature. It is something you're involved in, but it should not define your life.

You are a successful human being regardless of how your business is performing. I don't know you from this far, but I imagine there are a lot of people to whom you are very important. Those people rely upon you for the things you do that brighten and enrich their lives. None of those things have anything to do with your business. In fact, most of them probably don't even care that you run a business. They will love and respect you regardless.

Drop the idea that your business success – or failure – is in any way a reflection of you as person. If you don't, even if you *are* successful in business, you'll just spend your whole life paranoid about it. You will find that you're spending more and more time in the business, even though it is already successful, just to keep it successful.

You'll never be happy because you're always worried about losing it and concerned about how you would cope if that happened. Screw that. Business is a vehicle for living a great life – it does not define my, or your, life in any way.

My kids couldn't care less whether I own a business, work in one, or work for myself or for someone else. They don't care how many patients I've seen, how many buildings I've got, or if my Facebook ads are working. All they want is their bedtime stories read at 8PM each night and for me to ask how their day has been. Don't lose sight of what's important. All the money in the world won't fix a bad marriage or resolve a fractured relationship with your kids. These are the things that really matter.

The other way to overcome this is to, well, "get real."

If an employee screws up when you are away, that is great news. Why? Because it tells you where you need to train and improve. They're doing you a favor by highlighting a weakness in your business. You now know what you need to prioritize.

And if it keeps happening, it tells you who you need to replace.

And if you keep replacing people and the problem is still there, change your recruitment process or your training manual.

All of these are the real issues here. Once you realize that you and your business are not one and the same, you begin to let people do things for you, knowing that you're able to do things in your life that you couldn't if you didn't trust them.

Personally, I would rather my front desk person screw up a few phone calls than miss out on spending a week on vacation with my kids.

Wouldn't you? I love my business – *but not nearly as much as my kids*.

Trusting people means setting them free them to do their jobs without fear and allowing them to make mistakes they can learn from so that in the end they make the right decision consistently, regardless of whether or not you are there.

It also means that you might need to change your view on how you really think about people. Make sure you are coming from the angle that says most people are good and wanting to do a great job. Because they really are. Nobody comes to work wanting to do a bad job.

I've been around hundreds of business owners at meetings and seminars and many of them have a negative view of people firmly engrained in their beliefs as a result of being burned in the past. Yet, people are not all bad and they're not all out to get you or hurt you. Far from it. Most people are very good and decent. They want to help you and you have to believe that they will.

If you have a negative view of people – even a subconscious one – it *will* show up in your ability to trust your employees and lead them. That will determine whether or not you can set people free. And remember, all we're trying to do here is set them free so you can enjoy some freedom as well. Don't lose sight of this. There is an end to the means. They're there to make your life better.

Why don't you ease off a little and give them a chance to do it?

TRUST MEANS PEOPLE FEEL SAFE BEING VULNERABLE

A sure-fire sign that there's a lack of trust between you and your people is when your people push back at your new ideas. For example, if you're trying to raise rates, they'll tell you that they don't think people will pay, or that it is too expensive for your area.

What they're really saying is they don't trust *you*.

They don't feel safe enough to be vulnerable and risk the rejection that comes with a patient saying "no" to the new prices.

First, they worry that if they keep hearing "no," it will cause them to question their own self-worth. Second, they're afraid that you'll complain or, worse, fire them for being ineffective.

If people do not feel safe, they will not try new things.

They've got to be comfortable with you to even consider trying new things. Whether or not they will do this for you is really a measure of how they feel about you.

If you're asking them to do something new, they've got to know that you will support them and provide the appropriate training to make sure they can be successful. If they don't believe they'll get that, they'll push back and come up with a chorus of ridiculous excuses that you'll find yourself arguing over constantly. You'll always be scratching your head over why nobody on your team ever wants to try a new script or price increase. Even worse, you'll lose so much time trying to convince them.

Don't try to convince – just focus on making them feel safer and seeing it from their point of view. Don't focus on what they're saying – only why.

As I said in a previous chapter, the problem is never the problem. If people were able to understand their own issues and, in turn, be able to communicate we would all be better for it. Until that day, remember that what they're unhappy about is exposing something else. Much like we discussed in Chapter 2, if you spend time trying to figure out what that is, you'll have much more success driving change in your company.

HOW TO INSPIRE LASTING CHANGE IN YOUR PEOPLE

When you're getting more from your people – more than they could do on their own – you are inspiring change. It is a special attribute that should not be taken for granted. But it doesn't happen to every business owner and it definitely doesn't come automatically just because "business owner" is now in your title.

"I just can't get my staff to do things" or "no matter how many times I tell them, they never do as I ask" are just two of the things I hear private practice owners lament when it comes to their staff. The easy option is to think that this is a problem with *them*, that *they're* just too lazy to do what you're asking or that *they* have something against you.

But what if that isn't the case?

What if the reason this is happening is because of something that *you're* not doing, or that *you* lack? That thing is usually the ability to *influence*.

It is a quality that anyone who manages or leads people absolutely must have. You show me someone who can't crack the code on "people" and I'll show you someone who lacks the ability to influence. And given that you can't grow a business without having people do things for you, it's a vital skill to master.

We're only four chapters into this book and already it is dominated by the topic of people. People and leadership go hand in hand. Likewise, people growth and business growth also go hand in hand.

You could argue that the real business you are in is the people development business. And I often wonder if that is why so many private practice owners struggle to run a practice they are proud of – they simply don't acknowledge the importance of the people side of their business.

To have a chance of influencing your people, it helps if you are a fan of people in general. If you're skeptical about people from the get-go and you see your relationship with your people as transactional – as if they are units of production paid by the hour – then you'll never have a successful practice.

Sure, you can make money with a view like this. But, there's a difference between making money and *enjoying* making it.

Like we discussed in Chapter 2, *how* you make it must be considered, not just how much of it you make. It is much easier to make money – and more of it – if you have an influential relationship with your people. And if you want to be able to do that, there are three specific things required for you to be able to influence anyone.

Let's look at them in detail now.

1. Trust: Do They Believe You Are In It For Them?

In this case, the type of trust that we're talking about is whether or not your team thinks that what you're asking them to do has *their* best interests at heart. Any time you're asking them to do something, whether they express it or not, they will always want to know how it affects them.

Whatever the request, they'll want to know that you're going to have their long-term interests at heart. Is the new task you're asking them to do the start of a change in their role? Is it the diluting of their importance as you start the process of replacing them with another employee further down the line? Are you asking them to do things that don't fit the vision they had about their role at the company when they first started?

Are you asking them to do things that only ever seem to improve *your* position? If this whole thing is only about *you* – and how much money you want to make – there's no way they're going to ever trust that you are in it for them.

If they can't see the career progression that you promised them would happen, they'll begin to question pretty much everything you're telling them. And the moment that there's any distrust between you and an employee, they'll stop being as committed.

It is the same in romantic relationships, is it not?

If there's even a whiff of a lack of trust, one of the two in the relationship stops being as committed. What happens next? All sorts of second guessing about if the person is the right one, if they really love them, and the inevitable looking for problems that are always found. This wrecks any chance of a mutually fulfilling relationship.

Instead, it becomes a parade of heated arguments caused by insecurities brought on by a lack of trust. It exposes the worst side of each person. Twin B also shows up in romantic relationships. Twin A is who you dated and fell in love with. Twin B is the one causing the issues. If Twin B is present 90% of the time, you're in for a rocky ride in that relationship.

It is the same in a leader-employee relationship.

If either one of the two suspects that the other is not aligned with the values and vision they each hold, there's a disconnect and a breakup is inevitable.

As a leader, you must do everything you can to help your people see that their best interests are also being considered while at the same time getting what you want.

And yes, this is possible.

In this game, two people can win. The best relationships are the ones where both parties benefit and it's wholly possible in business. Maybe not in every situation in the short term, as there'll always be a time when someone doesn't agree with what is happening – but as long as both sides feel equally valued and respected in the long run, it can be achieved. In business, the marathon is always more important than the sprint.

2. Esteem: Do They Believe You Are Worthy of Emulating?

One of the things that you must have to be a great leader is some kind of "star quality" – something that your people want to inherit from you. It doesn't matter what it is, but there's got to be something about you that they wish they had.

One of the reasons for them to continue to come to work for you is the belief that if they hang around with you long enough, that star quality will eventually rub off on them and it will enhance or fill a gap in their own lives.

If there isn't something about you that they aspire to have, your influence is limited. It could be your high standards, your values, your confidence, or your beliefs or positive outlook on life. It could be how you live your life away from work, your relationship with your spouse or kids.

Whatever it is, there must be *something* they want from you other than just getting paid. If not, the relationship is purely transactional. It is about how many hours they work and how much you pay them.

Everything about being a leader is about getting more from your people. One of the ways that happens is by having something that you do, or that you represent, that causes them to want to step up and make a change in their own lives. You're influencing in a positive way and you don't even know it.

3. Permission: Have I Given You Permission To Coach Me?

This is huge. And, as it happens, this is nearly always where your relationships with your people break down. They may believe that you have their best interests at heart, they may believe that you have something that they'd like to emulate – but if the person you're leading has not given you permission to coach them, you've got no chance of inspiring them or making a lasting change.

And this is a big problem for us business owners, as many people are closed off from coaching. Many people are happy to accept what they've got or, as is more often than not the case, not even aware that an improvement can be made, never mind prepared to commit time to doing it.

Parents, and society in general, rarely do a great job of stressing the importance of being coached. Improvement is for life – not just the first 18 years.

Yet, the emphasis in that first 18 years is all on school and getting facts from teachers in order to pass exams. But there's little, if any, focus on how to become better at things once you've left school.

If school is about memorizing facts in order to pass a test (and mostly keep the government happy), then life is about *constant improvement* and *committing* to becoming the best version of yourself. To do that, you need to be coachable.

You must be willing to accept that every day is a school day, that there's always a deeper and more profound understanding of something – even if you think you know it all, you can always learn more.

Sadly, this isn't a philosophy most people carry with them.

Sure, they'll agree with you that this is the right way to live – but there's a disconnect when it comes to putting it into practice. This is a problem for business owners. It means even if you're a great coach – which anyone can be with the right training – you are still only going to be successful at coaching someone if that person gives you permission to do it.

Contrary to popular belief, leadership is not about commanding, evaluating, or standing over people to get them to do things. No. It is about communication, trust, respect, and feedback. All of these are a function of coaching.

The only real chance you've got at solving this issue is in the recruitment and hiring process that we'll look at in more detail in the second part of this book when we drill down into the role of the CEO.

INFLUENCING FRIENDS AND FAMILY: WHY IT IS SO DIFFICULT?

I speak from personal experience when I tell you that I've learned painful lessons on influence. If you're constantly at loggerheads with someone in your immediate family or circle of friends, as they never seem to listen to anything you're telling them, then what I am about to share might resonate with you...

In my business, I've never had that much difficulty influencing people. I haven't experienced many situations where people have revolted or pushed back at my new ideas and I've never worried about whether stuff will get done if I'm not there. It seems I've been able to positively influence many of the people who do come to work with me. That happens because of all the things I just mentioned.

Of course, there have been a few exceptions, but on the whole, by and large, I've been able to get things I've passed down to my team implemented. I've been able to positively influence my employees over a sustained period of time and rarely do I find myself questioning why they might not do the things I suggest.

However, in my home or personal life, I've *always* struggled to influence people the way I can at work. But when you think about it, it's very natural for that to happen. All three of the things that we've just discussed absolutely must be in place for you to be able to influence anyone, family included.

At work, you're more in control of the three critical factors of influence. This isn't the case with friends and family. It means when I sit with friends or family members and try to offer my advice on certain situations, it rarely ends well. I can have what I believe to be great ideas or solutions to their problems (that seem obvious to me), but they nearly always fall on deaf ears.

GET YOUR FREE RESOURCE KIT: PAULGOUGH.COM/LEADERSHIP-RESOURCE

I can recall countless situations where I would be talking to a close family member about a problem that they openly shared with me. After they told me the details, I would comment on the situation and make the mistake of advising them on what *I* would do – sure that they would go off and do it, or at least agree with me.

Of course, they never did.

(And why should they?)

I *used* to think that because I'd made a little bit of a "success" of my own life, it automatically meant that others would listen to me and follow my advice (like my staff do each day in my businesses). But that is not the case. Truth is, no matter how good I think my advice is, it rarely gets taken when it comes to family or friends.

Before I understood what was really required to positively influence someone (the three things discussed previously), this type of scenario was one of the most frustrating things in my life. I would spend all day at work with my team, asking them to do things that would yield results for the business, helping them in all areas of their own lives, and watching results happen there – and yet in my circle of friends and family, I couldn't get anyone to do anything. All of my efforts to influence would fall on deaf ears.

Has this type of thing happened to you?

Maybe it keeps happening to you?

Many business owners I speak to tell me it does.

And if so, it would be easy for me to just say "keep out" or "stop doing it." But I'm not going to do that. I'm going to ask you to look more closely at the three elements required to influence someone. When you do, you'll realize why it will just keep happening – why no matter how right you think you may be or how great your suggestion is for solving their problem, you'll be mostly be ignored any time you try to dispense advice.

Here's the reason: it could very well be true that they *trust* that you have their best interests at heart. It could also be true that they *admire* an area of your life that they aspire to achieve. But the chances of them being coachable are very unlikely. This is the most important factor in influencing someone and yet it is something you are unable to control.

During the recruitment process, I can pick and choose who I want to be part of my team, who I will spend all day working with and advising. In a recruitment situation, I can actively pick someone who is coachable. With our friends and family, we get what we're given. And sadly, most people are simply not coachable. It's harsh, but it's true. And I'm not sure you can coach someone to be coachable. This means that any time you're counselling friends or family members, your influence is severely limited. Doesn't mean you can't help by being a great listener – which is really want your friends and family want anyway – but it does limit your ability to influence any real change of the situation.

It can be frustrating, however, learning all of this was liberating for me as it really improved my relationships with the people close to me. I stopped getting frustrated when people didn't take my advice and I now just spend more time listening.

Of course, I still offer my suggestions as a way of doing the right thing by them – but I have absolutely no attachment to the outcome. It isn't about wanting to be right anymore. If they want to follow through on my suggestions, that is up to them. If they don't, that is up to them too. I'm cool with it either way. Whether they do what I recommend or not doesn't say anything about me and it doesn't even say anything about them.

Whether someone takes my advice or not is 100 percent out of my control and adopting this way of thinking is something that has really set me free from unnecessary moments of frustration or heated arguments with people around me.

I don't need to be right (well, not 100% of the time), and it doesn't mean I am undervalued just because my advice was overlooked. My ego always wants to be valued more. It always wants more attention and to constantly be right about everything. But I, Paul, have learned (and continue to learn) that feeding the ego is nearly always what gets me into situations I don't want to be in. I'm learning to override or at the very least delay it showing up in any conversation I am having.

Ok, we've covered a lot in this chapter. Let's sum it up. I will do so by reminding you that you are only as good as the level of your people and the standards they aspire to. You can influence them positively in a way that leads to lasting change only by setting a higher standard to show them what is possible. What is more, the simplest, yet most profound, impact you can have on someone is to *inspire their own change*. You can do that by believing in them and giving them the courage to learn to make mistakes while figuring things out – and, of course, a little of your time to help them improve and grow.

Alright, let's move on to the next chapter. This is a very interesting one where I'll talk to you about the four different types of leadership styles and let you know the one that you should aspire to have. Turn over the page and let's get into it…

LIBERATE DON'T ABDICATE

In the last chapter, we touched on the idea that your people need your support. You might be paying them, but they're still going to need other things from you – support being one of those things. However, there's a fine line between giving too much support and creating a culture of entitlement. A toddler needs support, but eventually she needs to be allowed to walk on her own. She has to be allowed to put her left foot in front of the right and if it doesn't keep up, she needs to learn to roll as she falls.

If her mother protects and supports her *too* much, soon enough that mother will end up with a lackluster teenager that soon becomes an entitled adult. That is not what you want in your company. People need support – but they also need to be challenged.

Support is about providing tools and information, plus coaching and training to allow people to succeed. It does not mean you give them everything or, worse, do everything for them. It does not mean that you give them an emotional umbilical cord to plug in whenever they need it.

That is not leadership.

That is what parents do who feel guilty about letting their kids struggle – and in doing so, they constantly deny their child the *privilege* of figuring things out for themselves. The struggle is real – and in many cases, it's very good for you.

After all, the difference between struggle and effort is simply a negative emotion about the thing you're doing. Remove the negative emotions that come with actually having to work hard or figure things out for yourself and you've got effort.

With enough effort, people are capable of achieving wonderful things.

It might feel nice at the time as you swoop in to solve the latest crisis or provide a box of tissues for the latest drama that has occurred in your office. But it isn't healthy in the long run.

It might feel nice to constantly be dropping and picking up your kids from soccer practice, but sometimes the best thing you can do is let them get the bus or figure out their own way there and back. If they have an iPhone, let them figure out the way home using Google Maps or help them get a paper route or a job at Starbucks to cover the cost of their own Uber. It'll be the best thing you can do for them.

Seriously, there's a very delicate balancing act between supporting and doing what everyone needs in order to grow – challenging them.

Highlight this next sentence:

Great people flourish in an environment that liberates and amplifies an energy that creates progress.

You get this by challenging people to be better.

When you challenge people, you liberate them. You set them free to figure out how to do things on their own and, hopefully, to do them better when you're not around to help. Is there anything better that you could ever do for people than this? To allow them the pleasure that comes only from accomplishing something on their own?

I see this in my six-year-old son, Harry, already.

We both love to build with LEGO. We've been doing it since I can remember. He used to want me to help him, but not anymore. These days, if I sit with him at the table to build a LEGO set, he's reached the point where he wants me there, but he doesn't want me to touch it.

Why?

Because he wants to be able to tell his mother that he did it all on his own. He does not want the accomplishment diluted by my involvement – so he builds it alone. I'm there *just in case* he can't find a piece or if the instructions don't make sense, but he will not let me touch his project. He is mostly trying to figure it out on his own because he wants to own the outcome. I'm there as a backup.

I believe this is how you should lead.

The phrase I like to use when coaching other business owners is, "Make things move, but don't touch them yourself."

If you analyze what this means, you will see it is the secret to successful business leadership. We want things done, but we don't want to have to actually do them ourselves. That is because if we have to keep touching everything, progress stops. Eventually we would touch too many things and we run out of time to keep making more things move. To keep growing we need ten things happening simultaneously, but we don't want to be actually doing any of them. It's when you're in a position where ten things are moving and you're not touching any of them, you're in charge of *growing* a business – not just running one.

GIVE YOUR PEOPLE THEIR OWN LEGO SETS

What we need to do with employees is give them the equivalent of the LEGO set. It comes with all of the parts you need, the instructions to put it together, and you and I are on hand to assist if there are any questions. But we must resist putting the pieces together as much as possible.

When you lead like this, you have a team that is independent of constantly needing your input. They should always know that they can get you – just like Harry knows I am there if needed – but they shouldn't need to be exercising that ability every minute of the day.

People are capable of achieving great things – but only if you give them the chance and you push them to do more than they currently think they can.

This is a recurring theme of leadership.

People are capable of many great things on their own – but with a great leader, they can be better than they ever imagined. Keep pulling people up to a level they don't know exists. Think about it: if they knew how to do it on their own, they would have done it already without you.

Of course, the idea of "supporting but challenging" does comes with a little bit of risk. What if you challenge people and they don't like you? What if they misinterpret your intentions and label you as "too pushy" or "overly demanding"? How do you deal with rejection if people interpret your intentions the wrong way? There wasn't a course in school on how to find the right balance between support and challenge, or making sure you're getting the best for your people. It is assumed that you get the best from them the minute you pay them. If only that were true. If it were, everyone would have a successful private practice.

As it stands, most have a private practice that relies too heavily on them being there every day, doing too much work when they are, and coming up with all of the ideas or ways to overcome challenges that crop up. And that is despite the owner having a huge monthly payroll obligation to meet and working more hours, often making less than some employees, and not able to get home for dinner before 8PM each night.

It's madness – but it's so often how it ends up.

WHERE TO START WITH EMPOWERING

Where do you start with this? Where do you start to make a shift toward creating an environment of liberation and empowerment? Well, you start at the very beginning. When an employee arrives in your world, it is important to start with high support before you get to high challenge. Support builds trust and without that trust you will never get people to be comfortable enough to be the best version of themselves.

But you must move quickly into challenging your people to be better in order to avoid a culture of apathy or, just as bad, one where your top people leave because they're bored and lack a feeling of accomplishment.

If you've ever had a scenario where your best employee leaves you – and you didn't really get a clear answer on why – chances are it was because they didn't get challenged enough working for you. It can happen more than you would like, so let's look at how to get this aspect of leadership right.

THE SUPPORT CHALLENGE MATRIX

Take a look at the image on the following page. It is called the Support Challenge Matric. It was developed as a model for leaders and coaches to help them pay attention to the amount of growth that was happening in their teams.

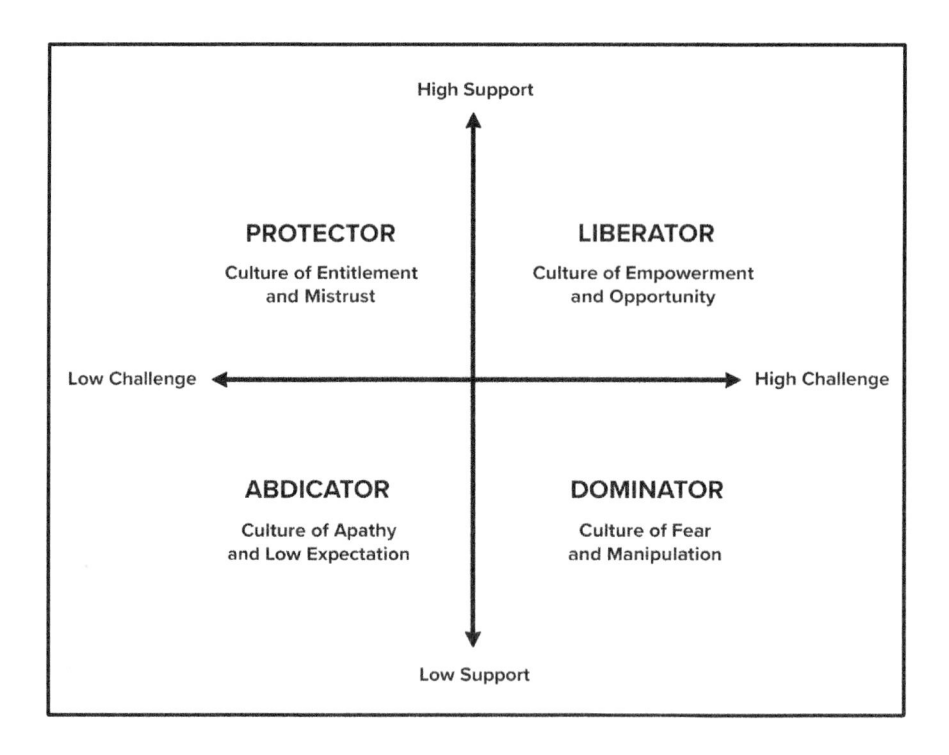

	High Support	
PROTECTOR Culture of Entitlement and Mistrust		**LIBERATOR** Culture of Empowerment and Opportunity
Low Challenge		High Challenge
ABDICATOR Culture of Apathy and Low Expectation		**DOMINATOR** Culture of Fear and Manipulation
	Low Support	

As you look at the matrix, understand that the leader your employees would want to follow and work for is a "liberator". To become this, you must spend as much time as possible in the far right hand corner of the matrix. That is high support and high challenge supported by a culture of empowerment and opportunity.

Instead of being a culture of high maintenance, aim to have your culture one of high achievement and performance through empowerment and providing opportunities for your people to grow. As a leader, you must become a liberator. That means you support your employees but simultaneously challenge them so that you set can set them free to be their best versions on their best days. Do this if you want "Twin A" to show up most days.

Let's take a look at all of the different quadrants that leaders can find themselves in.

DOMINATOR

When you're dominating, you are offering low support but the highest amount of challenge. You *expect* people to do be doing things instead of being grateful or appreciative of what is being done. You're asking your marketing assistant to start work on Monday and demanding that there's an influx of new leads by 5PM that same day – or else they're fired. You're asking a front desk person to book every new patient who calls – without giving them time to learn the scripts.

Your view is that you're paying people, so they should produce.

If they don't, they're a bad hire and they will be gone very quickly.

The difference between dominating and liberating is easy to define – dominators put their people under stress by requiring a lot of work to be done and expect things to be achieved with little if any support. Dominating leads to compliance, whereas liberating leads to engagement and progress.

Compliance may be an outcome, but because of the lack of support, employees perpetually fear disappointment, disapproval, and rejection when expectations are not met.

I'd say this is worst of all of the quadrants a leader could be in.

Yet, it is very easy for a business owner to land here, particularly if the business owner is from a successful family or is a serial entrepreneur.

The fear of financial (or opportunity) loss creates a low sense of psychological safety in the business owner. This causes them to become more dominant in the hope that it *forces* better or guaranteed results. The idea is that the more control or force you exert over the employees – even if it is only psychological – the more likely they are to perform for you. Yet, in reality, it works the complete opposite. The more control and force you exert, the more pressure they feel, the worse they are likely to perform. And because they don't perform, you try to exert more dominance. On and on this cycle continues and still there's no progress. The only thing that changes is the leader's blood pressure – it gets higher and higher. Results are short lived. Equally as short lived as most employees' tenures.

What should be pointed out is that you can move between the quadrants, often without even realizing it.

For example, if you're having a bad time at home or you're experiencing some kind of personal or financial challenge, then you could unconsciously move into the dominator quadrant. It's also easy for someone like you – who is successful – to forget that failure is a natural part of learning and growing. As a result, your leadership style shifts to being more about commanding and supervising instead of communicating and providing feedback on ways to improve.

The acute personal or financial duress you might be under makes you forego your usually long-term view of your business in favor of a short-term approach that demands results faster than is possible.

If you need the cash, you think compliance is the fastest way to achieve it. And if you're feeling a little crappy or suffering from low self-esteem, you think that getting stuff done – regardless of what that stuff is – will give you the relief that you're looking for. It's usually instant gratification that is often short lived, but it works for a few hours to make you feel better.

What is more, if you're feeling crappy, a way to instantly make yourself better (albeit temporarily) is to enforce some of the so-called "power" that you hold over people as their boss. Shouting at or being demanding of people makes you feel strong and good about yourself as you do it. The problem? It only lasts about a minute and then you usually feel worse.

ABDICATOR

When you abdicate, there's low support and low challenge. You're not really doing very much of anything. It's likely you've given up on your business or a specific person on your team and you're now tolerating their poor performance. Or, as is very common, you're too busy doing other things – like treating patients all day – to ever consider that your staff need help.

Abdicating is when you bring new staff into your practice, show them where the bathroom is, explain how to use the phone and computer system, and expect them to start booking in patients. If they're lucky, they'll get told about the policy and procedure manual from when you first opened the clinic (seven years ago) and they'll be expected to dust it off and figure out the best practices themselves.

If you're abdicating, you're ringing an outsourced marketing agency and telling them you want 25 new patients per week in return for their $2,000 per month fee.

You don't give them any direction, you're not willing to help them understand who the perfect patient is, and you're not going to be available for regular calls to improve the marketing message or contribute to the campaign. You think that since you're paying them money, you should get results and you'll check in a few months to see how they are doing. There's no support – and equally, there's no challenge.

When you're abdicating, you're turning to a recruitment agency to find a front desk person and you're accepting their offer to do it all for you. You sign the contract and that's it – they get to work on finding the hire you need. The next thing you know, a new front desk guy comes in to answer your phone and, in an instant, all of your problems are seemingly solved. That is, of course, until a few weeks later when you realize that new problems have been unearthed. The person they hired for you (absent of your involvement) was a cultural misfit (also known as a "pain in the ass") and has derailed two employees from doing the great work for which they were once dependable.

You now need to go back to the recruitment agency – but this time you ask them to find you three new hires.

You have to watch out for this happening to you. It can creep up on you all of a sudden with very little conscious awareness that you're even doing it. Becoming an abdicator could happen when you become overwhelmed by things such as recurring staffing challenges, cash flow issues, problems in your personal life, illness, or – as is nearly always the culprit – your case load is so full that you don't have time for your people.

You prioritize patients over your people and in doing so you often abdicate all of the other, often more important tasks required in the successful running of the practice. You're sure that the patients are more important and that staff will figure it out. You might be tired, bored, or burnt out, and that is causing you to abdicate your number one role –

developing your people. But whatever the cause, it is not the best way to lead.

If you abdicate, your people will wither from neglect and it's likely you will be left with a culture that is lifeless and has very low expectations. Making it through the day soon becomes the metric of success for your people and being successful or hitting outcomes is an afterthought. You'll see very little real growth in revenue and your staff will likely desert you after a year or so for a "fresh challenge."

In a culture that abdicates, there's no engagement or meaningful conversations between people. There's no people development and more often than not progress flatlines. It's very likely you have great employees waiting to step up to the next level for you – but their talents are not being put to use. They are screaming for direction and some of your time but they're not getting it. They're underwhelmed and their performance ends up being underwhelming. Yet, it could all be so very different.

PROTECTOR

In this quadrant, there is high support but low challenge. And here's something very interesting: as a health care professional, it's highly likely you will find yourself in the category of a protector. After all, that is who you are, is it not? You went into health care in the first place because you want to care for people, to protect them from harm. As such, that is in your nature. To protect is your natural tendency.

That is great for patients – but not for being a business leader.

Under this type of leadership, staff feel loved and protected most of the time.

The problem, though, is that protectors create a culture of distrust and disharmony. That is because they constantly let their staff off the hook for mistakes that keep happening. That is, of course, until the day comes when you've had enough of their constant mistakes – and you snap! You can't handle any more screw ups or constant forgetting of the process that leads to opportunities missed or problems created so your own Twin B – perhaps Twin C or even D – comes out and it isn't a pleasant sight. It definitely isn't you on your best day. It doesn't happen often, but when it does, everyone knows about it.

Here's why it happens: the protective culture you created lacks challenge, so disappointments and unmet expectations by employees are tolerated. First time is fine; second, third, and fourth are forgiven. By disappointments number six, seven, and eight you start get a little uptight. By nine you're on edge and then when the same mistake happens for the tenth time in a month, you let fly. It's like death by a thousand cuts. All of the little mistakes are stacked up and they build over time. Once it gets to a certain point, your resentment toward another mistake or a staff person failing at their job can no longer be contained. You let it out in a passive aggressive style.

You might be annoyed with them, but the real issue lies with you. The lack of consistent and timely feedback – as well as challenge – stifled growth and allowed mistrust into the relationship.

Here's an example that you might be familiar with.

After sixteen days in a row of your front desk screwing up the billing process that is now causing cash flow issues – and you letting her off the hook each time by apologizing *for her* and expressing how it's not her fault – you just let it fly. You on your worst day arrived in the practice and it wasn't a pretty sight. It was only thirty seconds of venting, but boy, did everyone know how you felt.

You go home that night, you reflect on what happened, and you feel bad about your actions and how you behaved toward your front desk.

The next day, you come into work and you apologize for *your* behavior.

Your front desk person is relieved. She sucks it up and thinks the whole situation was caused by you (not her screwing up for the sixteenth time). The employee feels as though she deserved the apology as she can't work out what she did wrong in the first place. After all, you tolerated it every other time she made a mistake. And that is where the distrust develops. That is where the inconsistency in the relationship creeps in. The minute you tolerate a mistake and you don't make it clear to them instantly that you will not accept it, the relationship between the two of you is built on a façade. It's a matter of time before a blowout occurs and trust is gone.

Life is very frustrating for a leader who is a protector. It is likely that you want everything to run smoothly and without any pushback. You most likely "hint" at what you want or use softeners to ask for it. But you don't do it in a way that is firm and leads to respect. You choose "nice" and hope to be liked instead.

Here's an example.

Rather than, "Okay, team, here's what I *absolutely need* from you all by the *end of the day*," you'll say something like, "Okay, team, if you happen to get a chance, it would be really great if you wouldn't mind doing this for me when you have time. If you can't, just let me know."

See the difference?

In the latter example, you're hoping to avoid any confrontation and choosing to use soft language that make it sound more conversational and you more friendly. Yet, that isn't how you lead. You don't need to be friendly or liked – only trusted and respected.

Leaders who favor protection often find themselves getting in the way of things being achieved. A culture of distrust is created because your staff are given so much support – with exceptions made in advance – that there's very little chance of expectations ever being met.

Here's an example. The operations mangers of my media and physio business are protectors by nature. They both see the good in everyone and everything. As much as I admire that quality, sometimes it gets in the way.

Whenever we would have conversations about the team they manage and the things individuals hadn't done – standards that haven't been met or targets not hit – both would often give me the reasons for why it was not done *in advance* of telling me it hadn't been done. Of course, when I say "reasons," I mean "excuses."

Examples: "Sally has had it bad at home this week and she hasn't done this or that" or "Bill is a little out of sorts because of his girlfriend issues and he missed the sales targets for last week."

The excuse would always come first and, unbeknown to both of them, they were protecting the employees from harm.

It got so bad that at one point we would often find ourselves arguing over whether or not the excuse was valid or if it warranted some mitigation as to why things weren't going so well for that employee.

Not so bad if it happens once in a while, but if that keeps happening you have to consider if the role is too big for the employee. If there's always an excuse, at some point you have to consider if the person is in the right role or they're simply not being challenged enough in the first place.

Allowing repeated poor performance can turn a potentially great employee into a perennial underachiever. It's vital you understand the difference and ensure that you're leaning more toward challenge than constant support.

When I studied this Support Challenge Matrix, I could see the situation so clearly. I pointed out to both of them that we have such contrasting leadership styles. I am very much in the liberator quadrant – sometimes I am too far to the right – and both of my ops managers are in the top left.

Now that we each understand it, I think it works really well when we come together to talk about the employees. Our contrasting styles force us to meet somewhere in the middle. If it were not for them, I would possibly be guilty of creating a "zero tolerance of excuses" company as I believe so much in people taking responsibility for their actions and what they eventually achieve.

If they're successful, it is because of them. If they're not, the same remains true.

I came to realize and continue to accept (struggling with it, but getting there) that not everyone can or needs to be at my extreme. The truth is that they really don't have to. They just need to be better than most at being held accountable – and the people who last in my organizations, are. Which brings me to the next quarter of the quadrant.

LIBERATOR

If you want to run a successful practice that you can enjoy owning, this is who you want to be as a leader – a liberator. If you study the definition, it means you will fight for the highest possible good of those you lead by intentionally mixing the amount of support and challenge as it is needed.

As a leader who liberates, you're obsessed with the people around you getting to the next level in their lives. It could be their personal or work lives, or both. It is a long-term commitment to your people that will not be achieved overnight.

It is a constant work in progress.

Being a liberator requires knowing how other people experience you – and then helping others discover the same conscious awareness of how they're being interpreted. To be a liberator, you need to have a certain level of sensory acuity – the ability to make good observations about yourself and other people – and you have to have a strong EQ (not just IQ) as well.

I believe that because the focus of society is nearly always on your IQ (school-type intelligence) and not on EQ (street smarts intelligence), people do struggle with leading others.

Often, people with a high IQ expect everyone around them to be as smart as they are and find it as easy to achieve as they do. But when the people they have to lead fail or underperform (in comparison to their high standards), communication breaks down and dissent is clear. If not careful, the leader with the great IQ soon starts to behave and act like a 12-year-old boy who has had his iPad confiscated.

Liberation of others starts with setting yourself free.

That means you getting very comfortable with who you are and being comfortable in your own skin. It involves rejecting social norms and outdated beliefs about how a leader acts and even how a leader looks. Jordan Belfort, as portrayed in *The Wolf of Wall Street*, might have shouted and yelled at his people, and he definitely wore expensive suits, but that doesn't mean all leaders have to look and act the same.

When I first started my career, I was in professional soccer. I wore a very casual "tracksuit bottoms and T-shirt" look to work most days. When I started my private practice, I continued to wear the same attire. Why? Because that is who I am. That is when I am most comfortable.

It's also possible that there is a little "two fingers up" to the business community who judge you on what you wear and how you look built into my decision.

I want to be judged for what I achieve – not what I wear.

I think I knew that very early on. Wearing clothes that I am not comfortable with in the office didn't fit well with me from the get-go. I've continued to wear shorts and T-shirts, a pair of jeans, or a tracksuit my entire business career. I own five companies, employ more than thirty people, own forty-plus pieces of real estate, and my companies generate nearly $5,000,000 in global sales. I've never worn a pair of fancy shoes to work in my life.

Sure, if I am on stage or at an important meeting, I will make an effort and bring out the shiny shoes. But I really only do that because I like to do it from time to time. I am making an intentional and deliberate decision. However, in my day-to-day running of the companies, I sit in my Nikes and athletic shorts from Lululemon.

Personally, I can't think of anything worse than having to run a company wearing a stiff suit and hard shoes. It would stifle every ounce of my creativity. I would lose twenty minutes every day actually getting dressed – not to mention the thinking time I'd lose each morning by deciding what tie goes with what shirt and so on.

I tell you this story because I think it's part and parcel of what is required of a CEO. If you want to set others free, you must first set yourself free. Don't be someone else's version of a leader. The confidence that

GET YOUR FREE RESOURCE KIT: PAULGOUGH.COM/LEADERSHIP-RESOURCE

oozes from a leader who is comfortable in his or her own skin — or shorts and T-shirt — is what starts the process of setting others around you free from social norms and outdated views.

By the way, I am not saying that because I don't wear a suit and someone else does that it makes me a better leader. Far from it. That isn't the point. If you want to wear a suit — go ahead and order the best you can afford and wear it like a Hollywood A-lister arriving on a movie set. But, what I am saying is that the first step to leading — to liberating yourself — is to be certain in yourself and not putting on a front to please others around you (who most likely will never be pleased no matter what you do). It's being intentional about what you are doing.

To liberate yourself from the shackles of other people's lack of thinking — their dogmatic and outdated philosophies — you must have a level of humility that allows you to accept that you have weaknesses yourself; to be okay with the idea that you don't have it all figured out. To understand and accept that you're a permanent work in progress. That despite your qualifications and the endless con ed certificates hanging from the wall, there's a bigger sign on your wall labelling your office as "under construction" that will never be removed. Ever.

This is a far cry from how most people approach their education and life's progression. It usually stops the day they leave school. Sure, there's a lip service paid to continuing education — in order to keep board certified — but there's no passion to learn or really grow. Why? Because they often dislike the feeling that comes from acknowledging that they don't know everything. The best leaders are the opposite. Their thirst for knowledge runs simultaneously alongside their commitment to uncovering weakness.

Weaknesses that, ironically, when uncovered and corrected, ensure that they become stronger and more committed in their pursuit to achieve.

GET YOUR FREE RESOURCE KIT: PAULGOUGH.COM/LEADERSHIP-RESOURCE

As a result, the ones who admit they don't know it all seem to get more than the ones who claim they do. How ironic.

As you grow as a leader, you realize more about yourself and that allows you to be a better leader of others. The best leaders have studied themselves first – they become aware of default patterns in how they respond to situations and continuously ask if that is the best way, hoping to find a better way.

When you have this going on for yourself, only then can you assist others in doing the same. In doing so, you liberate yourself from leading on autopilot and making rash, emotional decisions that often take you backward, not forward.

I guess what I am saying to you is this: the only option to liberate others is to liberate yourself first. Don't focus on how you manage others if you can't manage yourself first. You will never outrun a bad diet and you will never grow past a lack of awareness of yourself if you're trying to lead.

Okay, so those are the different types of leadership styles that you could adopt. In the next chapter, we're going to look at the qualities of great leaders. Some of those qualities might shock you as they're not the typical things you read about in leadership books.

Come with me to the next chapter and I'll tell you more…

WHAT ARE THE QUALITIES OF GREAT LEADERS?

Take a closer look at the best leaders and you'll find that they have something in common: a perfect combination of personal humility and professional will. It isn't just about having great work habits or being able to organize people toward achieving an outcome. There's often a modesty – even a shyness – about the best leaders who find themselves in a leadership position sometimes unexpectedly and often because of their determination and resolve to be the best version of themselves.

They can't handle mediocrity and they are compelled to achieve more than most because of the work standards that they set. It isn't about proving anything to anyone – except themselves.

The best leaders don't care what other leaders are doing (except if they can learn something from them). They care how they themselves are doing and how that is impacting the people they lead. There is a level of confidence and certainty that comes from within, often created by the actions that they take.

While everyone else is wasting time looking at what the others around them are doing – comparing – the leaders who are really leading are comparing themselves only against what was achieved yesterday.

Michael Jordan said it best when describing how he became the greatest basketball player of all time. I am paraphrasing, but he described how, in the aftermath of his first play-off finals loss, he realized where he went wrong.

He'd made the mistake of thinking that to be the best he had to be better than the rest. That may be true. But to be the greatest of all time, you have to be better than yourself if you're already the best. What a mind-set shift. At that point, you're not focused on anyone else. You're not losing energy worrying about what you lack – you're focused on what you need to do to improve. Big difference. One is scarcity mindset, one is growth oriented. Great leaders are growth mindset oriented and that is how their determination and resolve kicks in.

Let's take a look at a few of the qualities great leaders have in more detail.

1. Personal Humility

The best leaders are never boastful. They have a compelling modesty, often choosing to shun public adulation. It isn't about a pat on the back from everyone in the office – it is about a quiet beer or a glass of wine with colleagues to celebrate a collective accomplishment.

The leader is the one who is often rewarded by the public for results. But that isn't an accurate representation of what happens. The best leaders are rewarded in public for what they practice in private (often for years). The point is that the reward was *doing it,* not being recognized for doing it.

Of course, it doesn't always transpire this way. I am sure you can think of many great leaders who have become mainstream and do not fit this mold. For example – Donald Trump. He is a leader. Love him or hate him, he is a successful leader according to a lot of people's views of leadership. But to say that he is modest and displays humility is not open for debate. He simply doesn't offer either of those traits. Another example would be the late Steve Jobs of Apple. Depending upon the stories you believe or the interviews you've seen, it's possible to say that maybe he did not have compelling modesty. It's also fair to suggest that perhaps he did love to be rewarded by the public for his achievements.

The point is, though, how many Donald Trumps or Steve Jobs have there been in relation to the many great leaders you never get to hear about? There's always an exception to every rule, but for the most part the best leaders do not crave the public's attention or that of their team.

If anything, I think it's more accurate to say that Jobs and Trump are actually great marketers – doing anything they can to get their name and company recognized.

Let me give you another way to look at this. Take politicians, for example – they're often considered to be leaders of our communities (in principle).

Yet, the problem with many politicians is that they want and crave the public's attention. Most do not have compelling modesty, nor do they want to shun the public's attention. To get into the position in the first place, they have to do everything *but* be modest and shun the public's attention. The reality is that most politicians are the exact opposite of what it takes to be a great leader. I wonder if that is why so many of them lose their jobs every four years? Just a thought.

2. High Standards

I wrote at the beginning of this book that you do not need to have the biggest personality, nor do you need to be an extrovert, to be a great leader. That's because the best leaders act with a quiet, calm determination and rely more on inspired standards than inspiring charisma to motivate.

There's a time and place for the chest beating and inspirational speeches – but they mostly just make people feel good about themselves for a few minutes. When the chest beating stops or the speech ends, so does the motivation to do anything. That is why, as a leader, you must focus your efforts on raising standards. It is the only way to make a long-term and sustainable change to better the quality of your life or your business.

Candidly, if you look around in society, what you will see is a collection of people with what I would call "okay" or "average" standards. And for the most part, that is the type of life that people live. It is "okay." Could be better, could be worse. It is about average and on par with the other folks around them. What's more, I think most people would admit it, too.

A person's physical body is also a reflection of their standards. There's no need for me to ask a guy who is thirty pounds overweight what his standard is when it comes to his health – I can see that the standard is low. I can see with my own eyes that his standard for eating healthily is low and his exercise standard is just as low.

It is the same in the workplace.

I know precisely what someone's standard is for learning and wanting to progress in their career by the length of time they've been stuck in the same position. Anyone who has been in the same role for any length of time without any significant improvement in career progression has, whether they know it or not, set a low standard for their career development.

Some of this doesn't read nicely, but it is the truth.

Our lives are a reflection of the standards we set.

Same in business. It is about the standards that you and I set as leaders of the company. We might want to blame the government or the economic conditions in our town for a lack of revenue – but that is rarely true.

There's a business owner somewhere in your type of business who is defying the average. They're making more money or having more time with family – perhaps both. That person has higher standards for themselves how their business is run. The government and the low economic prosperity are the excuses that simply expose lower standards.

Remember, being a leader isn't just about inspiring. And it definitely isn't about your charisma. In a private practice, the financial performance of the company is a direct reflection of the standards set by the owner.

Sure, working for a charismatic boss might make employees feel better about themselves for a few moments as the boss announces the latest big idea – it might give everyone hope for a rosier future, but it will not ever be executed if the standards are missing.

Your inspiring charisma might open some doors for you, and it might attract some people to want to work for you, but it doesn't mean they'll continue to put in the work for you. Long-term success is about setting and raising standards. Let's get back to the politicians. Many of them are great when it comes to being inspirational and charismatic – but how many of them fail at the standards aspect of being a leader?

By the way, if you're picking up on an undercurrent of dislike for politics and politicians in my writing, you're on to something. I absolutely despise politics and the way governments have created a society that *thinks* they have to depend upon them. This is not a book for political discussion, but, it seems to me that governments are leaning more and more towards creating socialist societies and in doing so, breeding in people a state of perpetual helplessness. When the government underwrites and guarantees the welfare of everyone it means creativity is lost; it is no longer necessary as a quality required in each person's survival. Success achievement goes out the window in favor of a culture of entitlement. Thus, the system creates a class of people whose only creativity is to invent ways of milking the system.

And aren't they doing a good job at it?

I often wonder what society would be like, if, instead of taxing you 40% for making $100k, they fine you 40% if you *didn't*.

Just imagine how hard people would start to work and how creative they would suddenly become if they were actually rewarded for it – and not punished like the so called "fair" tax system does now.

Luckily for me I realized a few years back that politicians need us more than we need them. And, instead of making a decision every four years to vote for a party or person, I decided to "vote for myself" every day.

I've made politicians and political parties irrelevant in my life.

I do that by working on myself and focusing on the things I need to liberate me free from their decisions, at the same time helping others do the same. There are of course exceptions, but we need more independence from governments – not a wholescale dependence on them.

When you are free from ever worrying about which politician or political party is running the country, you really are free. It is liberating. You wake up the day after the election and the only thing you have to worry over is avoiding your neighbor across the street who voted for the loser.

That, and checking Facebook to see who thinks that even though their party lost, they still won it really. Have you noticed how politics is the only thing on earth where even when you lose – you can still lay claim to a victory? What a mess.

Anyway, believe me, whoever is your president or prime minister, they will never have as much impact on your life as you can on your own. Don't let anyone make you believe anything else.

3. Ambition Channeled into the Company

Something else that you will notice about great leaders is that they'll channel all of their ambition into the organization – not into themselves. They're obsessed with wanting the next wave of successful people in their company to step up and lead the organization. They've always got succession planning on their mind. It isn't just about what is in it for the leader, it is what can be achieved with or without the leader.

Great business leaders consider what would happen to the organization if the owner is not around – long before that is the case – and make succession planning a priority. By contrast, if you look at business owners who are more concerned with their own ambition, the focus of their companies is all on them and how the success of the company further enhances the leader's own opportunities and prospects.

Although I think that is very important, it should be a happy byproduct of the success of the company and those within it.

I think this is one of the biggest issues facing practice owners. There's a ferocious driving force called a "professional ego" that medical people have. It is as if our entire self-worth and identity is attached to our medical expertise.

It is that same professional ego that ends up running the clinic owner and, therefore, the company. It is the real root cause of why so many in private practice find it difficult to walk away from day-to-day involvement. The professional ego needs feeding, and that causes much of the focus to be on the clinic owner's own contribution and what he or she has done – not what he or she has assembled in terms of a great team.

But here's the thing I realized a few years back that helped me with this: fixing a patient's low back pain is impressive, but creating a team of ten therapists who each can do the same is something else entirely. It is next level. The impact is exponential. But because society does not consider this impact to be yours, it is difficult to embrace. Nobody really understands the skill it takes to assemble a team capable of helping so many people. They will acknowledge coaches of sports teams for creating great championship-winning squads, but the same applause is rarely, if ever, afforded to a business owner.

In my experience, they just assume that you are "lucky" for having so many good staff members. Seriously, people tell me this all the time. "Paul, you are lucky to have such great staff" is something my friends, family, and clients all tell me. I often respond with, "I know. I chose them!"

Still, the significance of the hiring process and onboarding is lost on them, not to mention the constant coaching that I am involved in.

But you know what? It really doesn't matter. The way I see it, you have a choice. Either my professional ego gets all the attention, or I walk away from it and give my family more of my attention.

If you're struggling with this, look at it this way: instead of helping fifty patients per week, when you build a team, you're now impacting 500 people per week.

Your impact is ten times greater.

That cold beer at the end of the week in a quiet bar on the way home from work all of a sudden tastes a lot nicer when you focus on this type of impact. Who cares if anyone else knows it? You do. Shouldn't that be all that matters?

It is when you have your ambition channeled internally – to be all about you – that you run into troubles with the clinic being tied to your every decision and every action. Fine, if that is what you want. But most don't. They want the professional ego "massaged" – but they also want to be able to leave the practice and one day have others run it for them.

That is like trying to go on a diet without giving up pizza or chocolate.

It isn't going to happen.

Focus on the bigger impact you can make by building a team that you're proud of. All of a sudden, being in treatment rooms becomes a roadblock getting in the way of achieving that. When you do this, it is much easier to resist the temptation to keep putting your name back on the schedule. You'll realize this comes at the detriment of all of the people you could really be helping by growing a team and letting those people take the praise.

They will get the thank-you cards and the nice gifts from patients. But you'll be the one who gets the internal satisfaction and fulfillment from knowing you made it all happen. Not to mention, of course, the autonomy and freedom of choice it brings to your life.

If you want to be a great leader, channel ambition into the people of your business and let them take the credit for pretty much everything that is good about your business. Use the leftover energy to really enjoy your life independent of what your patients – or extended family – may think of you.

As I always say, I loved being a physical therapist. But I love spending time at Disney World with my kids a hell of a lot more.

4. Take Full Responsibility

On the face of it, great business leaders are in a no-win situation. The high risk we take each day is rarely rewarded. That is because if it goes well, it is to your team's credit. If it goes wrong, it is your fault. You're going to spend the rest of your life publicly applauding your staff for the results of your company – yet, at the same time, publicly accepting their failings as your own. Great leaders reward their people in public and only get to criticize in private.

Which brings me to my next point: the greatest leaders look in the mirror to find the source of the problem.

However you look at it, every problem in your business is your fault. It is easy to look at the organizational chart and all of the names on there to allocate blame for the lack of results. And if you're ever tempted to do that, just ask yourself how those names got there in the first place.

Seriously, every problem you've got in your business is your fault. And you must live that way. It is liberating. When you live your life constantly blaming others for what has happened to you, or isn't happening in your business, you've given away your greatest asset – your power.

Look around you. Most people are powerless.

They're waiting for yet another politician to lie to them about their election promises and at the same time hoping for this one to be different.

They're waiting for their boss to give them a pay rise – even though they haven't contributed anything but years in the same seat to the growth of the company.

They're waiting for a handout from their parents, they're waiting for a husband or wife to change or do something to make them happy, and they can't see any way to be happy until that day arrives.

Basically, they're waiting for someone else to do something that will change their own lives and they're giving up their whole lives doing so.

You cannot do this. You cannot live like this.

As a leader, you must take responsibility for everything. Every time something happens that you don't like or didn't expect, the moment you take responsibility for it, you reclaim your power.

You might not like what is happening to you, but you can only change it when you own it. Even if it is just changing the way you see what has happened. This has been liberating for me and it significantly limits the level of frustration in my life.

If I take total responsibility, I can only be frustrated with myself. And that is difficult to do for any sustained period of time. If I am frustrated with my mother or father, or an employee or a close friend, it seems to last for a long time. I can mull over what they said or did for weeks on end and never seem to feel any better for it.

However, if I am frustrated with myself, I can't seem to do it for longer than a few minutes. That is because my ego won't let me. It doesn't like being wrong. It likes to be right – all the time.

So, by accepting that something is my fault, my ego gets to be right. "Yes Paul, you're right – you did screw this one up," says the voice in my head. When I confirm it was me who messed up, regardless of the circumstances, I can quickly switch from being frustrated at myself to looking for a solution to the problem I created.

When I do this, I feel better about the situation much faster. I also get my power back faster. I am in a position to tackle the next problem that I face as a leader head on, with a lot more awareness and clarity. And it is only when I have those two that I can change my focus and ultimately my actions. Without the latter, you've got no chance of getting outcomes you want.

If you are taking action and getting results, you also gather momentum. When you have momentum, guess what comes next? More great things happen, opportunity opens up everywhere you look, and people see that you're going places, so they want to ride along with you in the tail wind.

You become someone they want to follow.

They want you to be their leader.

You become someone who can get more from them and you're bringing a level of certainty to their lives that no one else can.

While everyone else is fighting and blaming someone else for their situation, you're showing people by your own actions how to get what they want, how to live how they want, and how achieve the outcomes that they couldn't get on their own. You're living proof of how to do the things they're craving to be able to do themselves. This is how you inspire people to lasting change – and it starts with you.

IS IT REALLY THE STAFF MEMBER'S FAULT?

Let's look at an example of how this works in your business.

If you employ someone who repeatedly makes mistakes, and one of those mistakes really hurts you, it is easy to say that it is that staff member's fault.

But is it really?

If someone on your team repeatedly makes mistakes, honestly, it is your fault. Not for employing them, but for *keeping* them. No one ever gets hiring right 100 percent of the time. There are way too many variables involved for that to happen. However, we can all get firing right.

They say you always get what you tolerate. In business, that is very true.

If you tolerate poor standards and you let your people make the same mistake more than three times, it is your fault and the only person to blame is the one staring you in the mirror each day.

The first time is your fault because you didn't explain it clearly. The second time it is their fault because they didn't do what you just re-explained. If there's a third time, it is your fault for tolerating repeated mistakes.

Whatever the situation is – it's your fault.

If the loan or line of credit you were expecting didn't get approved, why were you relying upon it in the first place? "That is what all businesses do," I hear you say.

GET YOUR FREE RESOURCE KIT: PAULGOUGH.COM/LEADERSHIP-RESOURCE

No, they don't.

Sure, many businesses do request loans and lines of credit, but they don't always do it because they are absolutely relying upon the loan to keep the business going. Many do so as a matter of preserving their own cash.

The simplest of rules when running a small business is to always have three months of expenses and operating cash on hand. How many violate that rule with their poor discipline – and financial standards – after a year or two?

How many business owners look at their checking account one day and decide they don't need the cash they've diligently saved up to that point?

Instead of being able to sleep at night on a comfortable pillow of cash, they spend it on "pimping out" their office with new computers or a new flashing sign out front. A week later, one of their biggest customers goes bust and the owner is in a cash flow bind.

Of course, they'll tell you that it was because they lost their best customer. They'll tell you life is a bitch and blame the recession or the stock market crash caused in China. What they won't tell you is that the couch you're sitting on in the waiting room is worth at least a week's worth of expenses and the TV that is on the wall is worth more than the marketing budget that could have been used to keep more customers coming in.

It is all about the *decisions* we make as business owners. The state of our businesses today reflects the decisions we've made in the past.

If you want to be a great leader, you have no choice but to accept total responsibility for everything that happens in your business. That happens when you have a level of personal humility that lets you live this way – in or out of your business. I always say that who I am at home is who I am at work. If I am humble and can display a level of humility at home, I will do it at work and vice versa.

Chances are you have both in your home life – you just need the permission to be the same at work. Permission granted.

5. Strong Professional Will

Next, let's look more closely at what I call the "professional will" of a great leader. This is the leader's determination or resolve to get results; to make great things happen whatever the environment.

If personal humility is about their personal standards and traits – this is about their *work*-related standards and habits that need to shine through the organization.

Great leaders are able to create superior results in whatever they're committed to or involved with. They'll make it happen no matter how difficult it appears or how many obstacles are in the way – or, as you will find out later in this chapter, what others might think of them. By contrast, weak or poor leaders decide to give up or get distracted quickly (and worry too much about what people think).

For a great leader, the challenge is the reward. For a lesser leader, the challenge or roadblock is an excuse to get distracted. All of a sudden, the fence needs to be painted, the grass needs to be cut, or an Amazon addiction needs to be fed.

Put simply, you can't be a great leader and not be able to produce results. You can't say you're going to do something and then not deliver the goods. Your team is watching, and you'll never be in a position for anyone to watch in the first place if you don't do what you say you will.

GET YOUR FREE RESOURCE KIT: PAULGOUGH.COM/LEADERSHIP-RESOURCE

Your work ethic and standards must inspire change in all areas of the business and your actual results must demonstrate it as well.

Even if you don't know how to do something, commit to learning, or find someone who can and hold them accountable to achieving the result that was promised.

This is a huge part of business leadership that I believe is misunderstood. Your job isn't always to "do stuff" (and it definitely isn't to "fake it until you make it"). It's common for people to judge you on how much work you do. On the volume or the amount of "hustle." But really, it's not about either of those two things. It should only be about what the company achieves.

Sometimes the best thing you can do as a business leader is find someone to do the tactical or low-level stuff that you've outgrown. And you need to be okay with giving that work up and knowing your job is to find more high-value work to do. But even though you've given it to someone else to do, you must remain on hand to make sure it is done and, crucially, in the required time frame. You must hold them to account. This is your real job and one of the highest value activities you can do.

To be a successful business leader, you need a level of tenacity and a will to succeed that leaves no one on your team uncertain about your level of intent to achieve success.

From the get-go of starting my business, I was intent on being successful. Failure wasn't an option. It was non-negotiable. Truth be told, it never even crossed my mind that my new business venture wouldn't work.

Sure, I was what I would describe as "cautiously optimistic," but I knew myself well and I knew I had the professional will to make whatever was needed happen. I was prepared to give up time and money. I would sacrifice almost anything to give my business a chance of being successful.

I look back now and realize that I was doing things that most people around me wouldn't ever dream of to improve the odds of being successful. I was investing in myself and my business at a level that was beyond normal. I was spending nearly all of the money that my physical therapy clinic was making on flights and trips from England to the United States to learn more about business.

I didn't just want to be successful "someday" – I wanted it to happen fast. I wanted my business success to deliver rewards that I could enjoy now. I've watched too many business owners toil for 20 years, hoping to enjoy the fruits of their labor in their retirement – but that day never came. I was adamant I wasn't waiting 20 years for success, so I decided to speed it up and I was prepared to spend money on speeding it up.

I've always believed in the value of coaching, so I decided to invest my money in myself – with business coaches – to speed up my business growth.

Of course, people started asking questions about what I was doing.

One of them was my accountant, who began to ask where all of the profit had gone in my usually very profitable private practice.

I tried to explain to him what I was doing with it all. I told him knew I had reached a roadblock in my understanding of business, the role models around me weren't at a level I aspired to hit, and if I wanted to get beyond them, I needed to learn more from people living at that next level. I knew I wasn't going to get better with time or experience. That isn't how it works. I knew the fastest way to get success is to get closer to people already having the level of success you want.

How did I know I had reached a roadblock? It was obvious. My income and my personal growth had flatlined.

I kept running into the same problems in my business and I couldn't get past those issues no matter how hard I worked. My standard was being met and I needed to raise it. Instead of accepting it or, worse, doing the same thing every day and expecting a different result, I made a commitment to myself (and my business) to figure it out. I decided to raise my standard. I realized that my personal growth would never exceed my investment in personal growth.

"I KNOW YOU WANT THIS DREAM HOUSE, BUT..."

Getting to the level I aspired to be at in business came with one or two awkward conversations and decisions. None more so that with my partner, Natalie, the details of a couple I'll share with you now and that you might find interesting to say the least.

It started with my desire to invest the $100,000 that I had saved – money that was supposed to be a deposit on our dream family home – on business coaching and mentorship that just happened to be in America. Try explaining that one to your partner and not being told to sleep in the spare room for a month.

Here's the full story.

It was 2013 and I had just become a father for the first time. My eldest son, Harry, had just been born and we were renting a beautiful home with a view to buying it. *I decided that it was not a good time to invest* in a family home – despite now having a bigger family. And what made it really difficult was the home was on the estate where I had *always* wanted to live. It was the type of home that my parents used to drive me by, and every time I wondered what it would be like to live in a "house like that."

Well, here I was on the verge of owning one and living on that estate with my young family, and instead of making the purchase, I chose to re-route the $100,000 deposit to business coaches, joining a few mastermind programs and heading to numerous seminars and events on the subject of business, in America.

At one point, it wasn't uncommon for me to leave the North-East of England late on a Tuesday night, fly out to somewhere like Houston or Philadelphia on a Wednesday, attend a conference for two days, and be back on a Saturday for dinner with Natalie and the kids.

I'd travel two hours in a car to the airport, fly 4,000 miles in ten hours through six time zones, get through immigration (often taking two hours or more), travel to the event hotel, attend the seminar, and then turn around with a book full of notes and do the journey all over again two days later to get back home.

Many times, I landed at 7AM and would be in the clinic at 10AM talking to my team about what I learned or in my office implementing what I had been shown. I was obsessed. My professional will took me to extremes that others didn't even know existed, let alone would have considered. Along the way I was setting and raising the standards in my office for others to aspire to.

I didn't know it then, but I was leading by what many would call "by example." They could see with their own eyes how willing I was to make the business work.

It was one of the most exciting times of my life and although I was jetlagged for most it, that first commitment to personal and professional growth was what really helped me figure out who I am as a person and a leader.

I believe the best part of being a business owner is in discovering who you really are along the way.

You get so many challenges and obstacles thrown at you that there's almost no choice but to develop and progress as a person. It's almost as if not wanting the challenge is the reason you're encountering it. You're getting tests before you've learned the lesson and, as such, you're developing your confidence and your resilience, all of which are contributing to your progress in life, making it easier to enjoy.

It was during this time that I got a completely new identity as a business owner. I was obsessed with getting new information and I loved how I felt about myself because of the decision I had made to grow and expand personally.

Ever since I made the decision to invest in my personal growth, I've lived with more visible purpose and energy. This means it is very difficult for anyone around me to compete with, or question, my professional will. I always say that if you're going to compete with me, good luck, to do so you're going to have to be prepared to give up some things that I know most people never will. That gives me an immediate advantage, but I really don't care if anyone is competing with me. I am in a fight only with myself.

Like Michael Jordan in the example earlier, I am not remotely interested in comparing myself to a business near me. Only myself. Me versus me.

Guess who will win?

As for the house we didn't get back in 2013…we waited more than three years, decided to rent a modest home for the time being, and had a second child in the meantime. In late 2016, we bought a house that was beyond our wildest dreams. One that back in 2013, we couldn't even have contemplated being able to ever afford – and what is now actually our second home.

That is because in 2018 we went on to get a residence in Orlando.

That is now our primary home and it happened as a direct result of the journey that I am on right now. The success of my private practice (that followed my $100,000 investment) allowed me the opportunity to start a second company helping others find that same level of personal and business success.

The point of that story?

When everyone thought I was crazy for investing in myself – for exercising my professional will – I knew it was only a matter of time before I could make the original dream bigger and better. Many people suffer from a ceiling in their thinking about what is possible. They're not able to connect their level of output – their will – with the quality of their life choices.

Lack of output, limited choices.

As a leader, you have to show your people. You can't just tell them.

I tell this story to inspire long-term change in you – so that you can inspire your people – and to show you that it takes a long-term commitment to improving your standards and your ability to run a business. But if you *do* commit, the life you can live is way beyond anything you can imagine right now.

My now three children live in a gorgeous little town outside Orlando (Celebration) and we have Mickey Mouse and Disney World in our back garden as well as a swimming pool and 300 days per year of sunshine. I play tennis every morning and I am able to walk home from work watching the sun set behind the palm trees on any night I wish. We have a beautiful lifestyle that once I could only experience on vacation for two weeks per year. Now I can live it with my family for fifty-two weeks of the year.

You might not want those exact things as a result of your leadership skills blooming, but I know you want something that resembles what I got: *the choice.*

"NATALIE, DO YOU REALLY WANT TO GO TO SWEDEN?"

Want another story of how I exercised my professional will muscle? Okay, you will love this one. And after reading this, I know you could be asking, "How does Natalie put up with him?"

Here goes.

It was back in 2013 again, just a few months before Harry was due to be born, that I asked Natalie if she wanted to come to London with me while I attended a seminar. She agreed. So far so good. She would hang out in the beautiful parks of London while I sat indoors and learned how to better run my business. She always draws the short straw.

Anyhow, I thought it would be nice to add another trip onto the week. From London you can get pretty much anywhere, so I looked at some cities I hadn't visited that we could reach in a short flight and be there and back in two days. It was the height of summer and we both agreed that Sweden would be a cool place to visit. So, we booked the flights. And the hotel. We would fly out after the seminar.

And it was all going so well.

That was, until I was shown some things about my business at the seminar that were so profound that I couldn't wait another minute to implement them. I knew I needed to get back to the practice and implement what I had just learned, or I would risk losing the impact of the ideas I was taught. That, after all, was what I had paid for and was looking to accomplish in the first place.

After the seminar, I asked Natalie how much she *really* wanted to go to Sweden and she said, "It's not on my bucket list, but I'd like to go." I said, "Okay, well, if it isn't that important, can we go another time? I really need to get back to the office."

Of course, she wasn't too happy with the decision. But Natalie being Natalie, she accepted it in support of my business ambition, and we went back home. I spent the next three days implementing a new marketing strategy (and a night or two in the spare room, again).

Of course, I am sure I was criticized by all of her friends and her parents were likely disgusted at my actions. However, two weeks later, I took Natalie to Dubai. And one month later, I took her to Italy just before the window for her to fly closed. I wonder what her friends and family thought about the holiday pictures she showed them.

The point?

Your professional will has to be so strong you're willing to do whatever it takes to get the work done. If you look at both of the true stories I have told in this chapter, they both involved my professional will taking over. It went into overdrive.

To many people, it would look like it is taking over my life. But thankfully, both Natalie and I see it differently. We have shared values, one of them being the importance of choice in our lives. Instead of taking over our lives, it enhances our lives because it *expands the choices available* to us in our lives and, with that, the quality of our life together.

Today's red wine is not nearly as important as the cellar full of it you're building by truly leading a great company and developing your business skills. With a cellar full of it, you can drink red wine every night for the rest of your life without worrying about if you have the money to pay for it.

To conclude this chapter, you must resolve to get it done at all costs.

If you say you're going to do something – do it.

Do not expect your team to get stuff done on time if you're not doing the same. Make it impossible for them to lower their standards because you lowered yours. I am not saying be as extreme as me, but you must find your own level and it must be above that of the people around you.

Okay, let's move on to Chapter 7, where I'll help you develop your own leadership philosophy. This is akin to you writing your own "profile" and telling anyone who is interested in coming to work for you how they can expect to be treated. I'll help you develop your own by sharing mine. Turn the page and let's get into it!

DEVELOPING YOUR OWN LEADERSHIP PHILOSOPHY

If one of your top jobs as a business leader is to help your people be successful in their roles – to influence them – then one of the most important things you can do is align them with your leadership style. If you can't align with your people, chances are the operational or clinical skills that your employees have will make little if any difference.

As an example, we've all witnessed superstar football players – who possess great technical skill – fail to perform for a particular manager or team. The reason is *not* that either is bad at their respective jobs. The reason is that the two are not aligned. How the player likes to be managed and how the other likes to do the managing do not match up. For a partnership to be successful, you need both. And preferably the two are considered before the employee starts.

It is common for managers to ask in an interview, "How do you like to be managed?" It's a great question to ask. However, it is very rare for the manager to clearly spell out *how they manage* or *what their style is* so that the employee can make a decision on *them*. In an interview, it isn't just about you interviewing them. The potential employee is also interviewing you.

During interviews with potential employees, I make a point of showing up as the person who will be leading them. I make a point of *not* arriving to the interview trying to be a nicer version or a different version of the guy who they will work with each day. I actually try to go the opposite way. I lean more into the leadership style that they'll see day to day to give them an accurate view of who I really am.

I've always believed that as much as I am interviewing someone, I too am on trial. Great candidates are not looking for jobs – they're looking for a place to call home. They're looking for careers and to work for people who can help them achieve more than they can on their own.

I do not want someone agreeing to work with me because they liked the nice guy who did the interview but then realize later that I am completely different. That wouldn't be fair. It wouldn't be congruent. It would be as if they were interviewed by a total stranger. It is a fake way to live and yet so many business owners do it.

There's only one way to live and that is true to who you are – always.

If in doubt, err on the side of being a slightly more candid and assertive version of yourself so that there can be no doubts about who they'll be working for. I turn up for an interview a few minutes late – on purpose. I want to see how they react. Do they take it personally? I have been known to use colorful language during an interview – that's because I occasionally use that same language in my day when I get passionate about things.

To be clear, not when I get angry.

That rarely, if ever, happens.

But I do get passionate and animated about my business and my language often changes. It is never aimed at my employees – ever. It is a conversation I am often having that sees my energy naturally rise and my tone shift with it. I get very excited about business and occasionally you'll hear it as my language changes. It isn't a habit – it is a reaction to a change in my state and how I am feeling.

The reason I choose to use occasionally colorful language in interviews these days is because I once had a front-desk person in my physiotherapy business who quit after two weeks – blaming my language. She called to hand in her resignation and explain she didn't want to work for someone who cursed.

Now, the truth was this: she was dreadful at her job and she was about to be fired anyway. She jumped before being pushed and used my language as the smokescreen to hide the fact she couldn't follow a basic procedure.

But after she said what she did – that she did not want to work for someone whose language is occasionally colorful – I thought long and hard about it and decided to change.

From then on, I made a point of cursing during interviews.

I do it at the same point every time – just as I am passionately describing the company and my future plans for it or, as is often the case, dismissing some outdated view people often have about what it takes to be successful in business.

I do so to make sure that they know who I am. Not a guy who curses at people – but one who gets excited and animated about his business and, as a result, becomes a little less selective about the words he uses.

Basically, who I am is who you will see in the interview.

If you don't like the fact that I passionately curse – don't take the job.

I've got more than thirty employees – many of whom have worked with me for ten-plus years – who don't mind it. In fact, many actually say it is what they like about working for me – that I am passionate. That I have an excitable, youthful energy that is infectious and that you would want to be around.

I am not for one second suggesting that everyone likes it – and that is fine. But here's what I say to that: don't work for me.

If you're that sensitive to words that you've probably used yourself many times, then don't come to my workplace. I make zero apologies for being passionate. And if I have to consider my language around grown adults, it will curb my passion. Take away my passion and I'll not have the business to employ people in the first place. It is easier to be clear about who I am from the get-go and then let the employee decide if they like it or not.

I would describe this as being authentic – and it is just one example of the many things that I would have under the banner of *my* leadership style. To say that I am passionate about growing my business is an understatement.

Likewise, I am equally very respectful.

In more than a decade of managing people, I have never once sworn <u>at</u> an employee and I can count on less than two fingers the number of times I've ever even raised my voice to an employee. That isn't my style, primarily because I take ownership of almost everything that is wrong in the company that might lead to me becoming angry in the first place. What would be the point of getting mad? I would be doing so at myself and that is just dumb.

GET YOUR FREE RESOURCE KIT: PAULGOUGH.COM/LEADERSHIP-RESOURCE

Don't get me wrong, I can very quickly get to another level of frustration or angst because of poor results. And you'd know about it through the intensity of the tone of my voice and my body language would inevitably change. But I rarely if ever really shout or get vocally aggressive in the way that so many business owners do – sometimes daily.

If you're wrestling with developing your own leadership style, my best advice is simple: be authentic. Don't be someone you think people want to see – that is fake, no one wants to follow fakes.

Be true to yourself. *Be respectful to people and their individual situations, be kind and generous with your time, and be fair but firm.*

And don't forget to be fun with it all.

Business doesn't always have to be so serious. If it is, you're doing something very wrong. Fix that.

Those are the qualities that all good leaders must possess. After that, it is open to you and how you want to lead. What is more, make sure that all of your decisions are conscious ones. Don't do things or say things or behave in a certain way without being aware of it. As you evolve as a leader, you evolve your leadership philosophy. There might be things you did ten years ago that you wouldn't do today.

In the same way, there should be things you do right now that you won't do in ten years' time. Your leadership style is going to be fluid. The more you learn about yourself, the more that you'll adapt. The more mistakes you make, the better you'll become. The more experiences you have, the stronger and more confident you'll become.

Fail forward with your leadership and eventually you'll look back and realize how far you've come. If you're on a journey to be the best version of yourself, you want your employees telling you how you've changed over the years. To suggest that you have to have it all figured out now is not being fair to yourself. You're just trying to satisfy your ego if you think that way.

Remember, as a leader you're still going to be led.

You're still going to be influenced to improve your own standards and become more certain. Because of this, you will evolve, and you will grow. As you grow, you'll pull everyone up around you and, in the end, you'll realize that as you grew as a leader, so did the people around you.

By definition – you're leading.

PAUL'S LEADERSHIP PHILOSOPHY

To help you develop your own philosophy – to be certain in who you are and how you will show up every day – here's more on how I work and what I expect from my team. This isn't for you to copy verbatim; it is just to stimulate your thoughts about who you are and how you might define *your* leadership style if someone were to ask.

I've written the rest of the chapter as though I was writing it to one of my employees or a potential new hire. It wouldn't be a bad idea for you to create your own version of this and then give it to all of your team. Here's how mine would go.

MY STYLE, IN GENERAL

- For the most part, you'll find I'm a very relaxed guy. Very little bothers me and I'm very good at keeping my emotions in check. If I am unhappy, I wait for specific times in the day or week to bring it up. That is a problem for some people. Just because *I* am relaxed, it doesn't mean that my *standards* are.

- I am very open and straightforward – what you see is what you get. I have not got time for games and I do not come with any hidden agenda. I say what I mean and there is nothing to read between the lines. If I say you're doing a great job, you're doing a great job. If I say you can do better, or I challenge you to do more, it means I think you are letting yourself down. It is a compliment. I am reminding you that you are better than what you're doing right now.
- I am *very* impatient. It is the reason you're employed now and not in five years. I do not believe patience is a virtue – it is often an excuse to underachieve.
- I am at times unreasonable. Scrap that, I am unreasonable more often than not. I am unreasonable in that I refuse to accept being told that something can't be done. Again, you are here today – in this job right now – because of my repeated and never-ending unreasonableness. It is possibly my greatest attribute.
- I am not a fan of people being "busy." Ants are busy – but they don't achieve all that much. They're largely pointless. I am outcomes and action oriented. Fair, but somewhat impatient. I value the outcome being achieved and abhor excuses and rationalizing of why something could not get done.
- I like to know the bad news. Do not keep it from me. If you smile and tell me everything is going well and I find out later, you knew it wasn't, then there's a level of distrust being created between us and it is difficult to repair. If you know something is going to affect the company, tell me before it does and I'll be able to deal with it better.

- Contrary to that, occasionally I will vent about something I do not like if something has gone wrong. If you suspect I am venting, that I am being completely irrational, or you've caught me at a bad time, take everything I say with a grain of salt and ask me a day later what I really think. You'll nearly always find I have a different perspective.

SOMETIMES WRONG, RARELY UNCERTAIN

- I make very quick decisions. I may take my time to decide – to think – but when I have made my decision, things happen fast. *It is often the case that I am wrong, but I am rarely uncertain.* If you have a feeling that I am wrong, you'll need to let me know that very quickly. What is more, I am very happy with you telling me that I am. I will thank you for it.

MY BUSINESS PHILOSOPHY

- It's always about providing maximum value to our customers. I want customers for life. I do not want to get a customer to make a sale. I want to make a sale to get a customer to enhance and add value for the rest of their life.
- The source of all value in any business comes from my staff – that is you. You have a big responsibility. I believe that the value does not come from the product or service – that is what the customer gets in exchange for paying their money. For the most part, they don't want products or services – they want to *feel* a certain way about getting them. That is value and you deliver it by providing superior customer service, going over and above a typical

employee-customer relationship to build lifelong relationships with our customers.
- Employee relationships are the secret sauce to a great culture. If I don't have a great culture, my clients will not have a great experience and maximum value will not be felt.
- I strongly believe in the customer service experience, in helping customers decide what is right for them – not the other way around. The fallacy in business is that the customer knows best. In my experience, that is rarely true. It is why so many people buy things they don't need or never wanted. Our job is to never compromise our most important role: helping people make good decisions about our products and services.
- I believe in accountability. I do not know anyone who has ever achieved success without being held accountable to higher standards. I am held accountable in many areas of my life – and that is another reason this business exists. Individual responsibility (ownership) is essential and it means that individuals will be responsible for their own results.
- My responsibility is to establish the major outcomes needed for the business to be successful, set the priorities, and ensure that you have the resources you need to achieve goals. Your key responsibility is to deliver the outcome and get the results we agreed upon in the time frame we set. You will have a lot autonomy and complete accountability to succeed. My job is to ensure you have everything you need to succeed – your job is to not let yourself down.
- You are compensated on the twenty-eighth day of every month for your help in achieving the outcomes I decide I want for the

business, and in the fastest way possible. What I want is not open for debate. How we achieve it is.

- My business is my first baby – I care about it nearly as much as the other three I have. I'll do anything to protect it and ensure that it grows old. I do not expect the same level of intensity from you, but the closer you can get, the better. Give it the same love and affection that you would give to your niece or nephew and we'll get on fine.

- I have very strong opinions. Success as a leader requires strong opinions on important matters, but you and I do not have to agree completely. I have hard and inflexible rules about what is good, what is acceptable, and what is stupid and sloppy.

- Consistency is important to me. I work to ensure that I show up the same person each day. You will rarely see a wild side of me, and you'll hardly ever see a negative side. I am for the most part pretty consistent in my actions and emotions. I am definitely a glass half full person, but at the same time I not an eternal optimist who loses sight of reality.

NEVER OVERPROMISE, ALWAYS OVERDELIVER

- Never overpromise me, your colleagues, or our clients. But feel free to overdeliver.
- If you tell a client you will do something, do it.

LEAVE YOU EGO AT THE DOOR

- The fastest way we can get stopped in our growth is if our people stop communicating. You might be in marketing, but sales and finance still need to know what you're doing. You might be in clinical care, but the marketing team still needs to know what our clients are saying. The better our communication, co-operation, and support, the faster and farther we will go.
- Improvement is integral to fulfillment. The most fulfilled employees are always the ones who are committed to getting better. If you're committed to getting better, success will follow.
- You might be in a senior or supervisor position – you might even be a medical professional – but you don't bring your ego to work. Check it at the door. We have different levels of responsibility, but we're all equally responsible for achieving the business outcomes. Do not ever feel like you're inferior and never make someone else feel that way either. The latter is not tolerated.

EXECUTION MATTERS

- Good ideas are easy to come by. Candidly, I come up with dozens every hour. But execution is where the magic happens.
- Excellence requires good ideas to be well executed. Do not leave your contribution to the company at the idea phase. Good ideas must be whittled down to the top one or two best ones and the most important to execute.

MY EXPECTATIONS OF YOU

- High performance – all of the time. We are a numbers/outcomes-based business and we must produce the results we agreed upon.
- Back me in public, criticize me in private.
- Support the decisions when they're made. You will be invited to contribute before those decisions are made. Nothing is worse than someone who sits silently during the decision-making process and then, after the fact, seeks to undermine the decision made.
- If you have a hang-up about anything, come to me personally. If you are not happy with me, tell me in private. My door is wide open to criticism.
- If you're not happy with a decision, make sure you have an alternate suggestion. If you're not armed with an alternative, you're moaning. I will not tolerate moaning.
- If you tell me I am wrong, you must tell me how to improve.
- Agree to not know enough – but commit anyway. It might be that you don't have all of the facts. That is okay, I rarely ever do and yet we've got this far this fast. Agree to fail forward and commit to filling in the blanks as we discover more.
- I hate anyone saying, "I didn't have time." One of my pet peeves is being told a day after a project was scheduled to be completed that someone ran out of time. I accept that you might run out of time. But I want to know ahead of time it is going to happen. Otherwise, you simply forgot. If I know you are pushed for time, I can help you reprioritize and remove other projects from you that are getting in the way. Tell me you're running out of time – but don't tell me you did.

- Do not tolerate me putting more and more on your plate. I am an entrepreneur at heart. I am used to spinning many plates without dropping them. I do not expect the same from you even if I keep giving you the plates. You have permission to remind me that if I keep giving you more plates then you can't do your job.
- Plan your day before it starts. Your workday must start with careful consideration of what you need to achieve that day. Ideally, you did that the night before you arrived for work.
- Prioritizing is the number one skill of any employee. If you can't prioritize, you're working hard on the wrong things. Every day starts with prioritizing the four to six major things that must be achieved that day in order to help you achieve your goals for that week and that month. Anything else is busy work. Remember, ants are busy – but they don't achieve much.
- Help others. You're not just paid to do your own work. You're paid to be an influence and helping hand to team members who need it. Check in regularly with your colleagues to see what blanks you might be able to fill in for them. Hallway conversations are perfect for this. "What are you working on?" is a great way of keeping lines of communication open across the company.
- Leave your problems at home. We all have problems. And we all think our problems are the most important. They're usually not. The workplace I created is a place to come to forget about things happening at home. It is a nine-hour break from things going on at home.
- Tell me when you want to leave. The reality is that I'll know three months before you tell me that you want to leave. It will show up in your performance. On the off chance you've not dipped in

performance, please tell me that you want to leave as early as possible – even if you haven't yet found another job. I promise you that I will respect you more and honor your employment until you leave. The more time I have to replace you, the better chance I have of finding the best candidate for your role.

- If you're on time, you're already late. The time sheet says 9AM, but if you arrive at 9AM, then you're not starting work until 9:10. If you do that every day, you've taken nearly four hours of unauthorized paid leave every month. That isn't fair. Equally, if you leave the building at 5PM, you clocked off at 4:50PM. That is another four hours of unauthorized paid leave. You're now claiming a day per month. That is twelve days per year. Nearly two weeks of productivity lost in my company. Small cracks lead to broken windows.
- Be coachable. My organization is dependent upon you being humble enough to accept that you don't know it all and hungry enough to want to know it all.
- In summary: do the right thing. Be humble, be hungry, and be smart. Show others you care and be coachable.

CALL IT TIGHT

- Say what needs to be said, when it needs to be said, to whom it needs to be said. If your colleague needs to be reminded that work starts at 8:50AM, not 9:00AM, please tell them.
- Equally, if your standards are slipping, thank your colleagues for reminding you that you're letting yourself down.

- If someone – me included – calls you out for your lack of performance, your first instinct might be to wonder why you're being criticized and begin to defend yourself. Take a beat and realize the person calling you out is most likely just fed up with you not doing something you said you would, or that is part of your role. Thank them for it – they're giving you a chance to put it right and save your job.
- If you make the same mistake twice, more fool you. If you make it three times, more fool me.

MAKE MISTAKES, BUT DON'T BE RECKLESS

- Be courageous and adventurous, but don't be reckless. I don't want a risk-averse organization. At the same time, I cannot tolerate recklessness. Be guided by your intent.
- Learn from your mistakes and, even better, keep a log of the lessons you've learned from the mistakes you've made in the pursuit of progress. If you stop to think through all of the consequences of your actions, it is possible that you will make a mistake, but it will not be costly or irreversible. The key is to *think*.
- If you make a genuine mistake that a client does not agree with, I will always back *you*.

ONE-ON-ONES

- I manage by a lot of walking around and I talk to all of the staff about how all of the other staff are doing.

- If you feel you need to talk to me, I welcome it. Please have an agenda and send it to me twenty-four hours in advance.
- If you feel you could do with or benefit from my insight, experience, or advice on any topic – personal or work related – just ask. Always ask for a meeting with me if you have a cultural or communication issue that is unresolved.

IMPRESS ME WITH ACCOMPLISHMENTS AND RESULTS

- Do not impress me with what you plan to do – only what you *did* do. Do the work to be successful in your job, but don't expect a pat on the back for how many phone calls you made or emails you sent.
- If we have a meeting, plan for it the day before. Have an agenda with the three things you'd like to discuss and possible solutions for them all. If a meeting is worth having, it is worth planning for.
- If someone from outside wants to meet with you, demand the same. You want an agenda and the three possible outcomes, or you don't show up.

So there you go, my leadership philosophy and style. It's there to provoke thoughts about your own so that you can be clearer and more confident about who you are and how you will lead.

I find that the more awareness you have about who you are and, in this case, about how you want to lead, the more certain you are about doing it. Indecision kills any chance you have at being a successful leader.

A business leadership philosophy is a living, breathing, and ever-evolving document that describes who you are. Refer to it any time you're feeling a little lost or your leadership style is being questioned. It might just do the job of reminding you who you are and what the purpose of this business of yours is in the first place.

It certainly isn't to please everyone – which is usually what you've done any time you find yourself questioning your style or having doubts about whether you're a good leader.

That's the end of Part 1. Well done for getting this far! You're doing great.

So far we have looked at general leadership skills and attributes as well as the difference between managers and leaders. You've come a long way. In the next part of the book, we're going to look at business leadership – and the specific role and skills required of a CEO.

Come with me, you're about to be enlightened!

PART 2: YOU, THE CEO

To fully understand the next part of the book, please download your CEO Job Description and Scorecard here:

www.paulgough.com/leadership-resource

WHAT PHASE OF BUSINESS OWNERSHIP ARE YOU IN?

Take a good look at private practice owners. How many would you swap places with? Probably not very many. And yet there will always be one in your town with whom you would. That is the one with the best business skills.

Businesses don't run themselves and sadly most business owners don't know how to run them either. Business failure is more often than not the result of a bad business owner – not a bad business. Business owners who are successful get there because they know how to run the business end of their business. They know how to create sustainable financial success.

Making money is one thing – making it over a sustained period of time is something entirely different.

How do you spot a business owner short on business skills? They typically spend years jumping between working longer hours and getting better clinically in an attempt to grow their business.

When the Facebook marketing strategy they pieced together in an hour flat doesn't work, they revert back to chasing doctors for referrals or enroll in another clinical skills training course, hoping another CEU accreditation will improve their cash position.

Neither plan worked the last twelve times they tried them, so chances are they won't work this time, either. They're trying to solve a strategic problem with a tactical solution. It never works.

It's also why so many business owners are largely tired and frustrated when they want to be free and rich. If you want to be free and rich, maybe you need to get a better boss?

(Ideally, one with better business skills.)

Here's the blunt truth: it *isn't* the horse that wins the race – it is the jockey with the best skills. It *isn't* the driver with the fastest race car that wins the race – it is the one with the best skills. Somehow, somewhere, this concept has been lost on private practice owners who have been schooled by a system that kneels at the altar of clinical skills, believing the only way to be successful is to be the best clinician you can be. That is very true if you want to be a great clinician, but if "business owner" is now in your job description, then the skills you learned at PT school are redundant.

You've got a new job now as a CEO (or aspiring CEO) and there's a new set of skills to be learned to do it right. Being good at diagnosing sciatica is very different from diagnosing a cash flow issue or a culture problem. It's the likes of the latter that you're going to need in order to be a world-class CEO of a profitable private practice.

SO HOW DO YOU BECOME A BETTER BUSINESS OWNER?

However easy they may make it look, great business owners are not born with business knowledge. Much like great golfers are not born with a great golf swing. The successful ones study, practice, and master the art of hitting a golf ball from a very early age. You could give me Tiger Woods's golf clubs, his caddy, and let me have a ten-shot head start, but if I don't have his skills, it won't make any difference – he will still beat me over the course of 18 holes.

You could give me the fastest F1 racing car – but it won't make much difference as Lewis Hamilton will still beat me. Why? He has the driving skills. You will never beat the person in any field, in any sport, in any business, who has the best skills.

Sure, you might beat Roger Federer once if he's having a bad day (a very bad one!., but over the long run, Roger Federer will beat you enough times to win more trophies than you. That's because he has the best tennis skills.

The same is true in business. Business skills are the foundation for long-lasting business success. And that's what the second part of this book is all about. I am going to introduce you to some of the specific skills you need to home in order to become a successful CEO and business leader (as well as the daily tasks you should be focusing on, so you better prioritize your time).

And it will be worth it for you. The juice will be worth the squeeze. The value created from having great business skills and constantly honing those skills will far outweigh the value created by constantly treating patients. If we're judging value on the time, freedom, money – and choices – that you've got in your life, then it is undeniable that refining your business skills will add more value to your life than anything else.

GET YOUR FREE RESOURCE KIT: PAULGOUGH.COM/LEADERSHIP-RESOURCE

Even if you tell yourself that you want to impact patients, consider this.

On your own, your clinical skills will impact 20 to 25 patients per week. Grow and scale a successful business that employs five physical therapists and you could impact more than 100 patients per week. If you want to help people, could it be you *owe it to the people in your town* to be the best business owner you can possibly be in order to impact more of them? Just a thought.

We all have different reasons, but the ultimate reason I wanted "business owner" in my title is because it allows me to live an autonomous life. Being a business owner, I get to be independent in my thinking and in my actions.

I get to choose how my day looks, when I start, when I finish, when I travel (and for how long) and even where I choose to live. I left England to live in the United States simply because I got fed up with the cold, dark, and damp weather interrupting my enjoyment of the simple things I love to do with my kids. It's hard to enjoy going for a walk along the beach or being at the play park when it's always raining and cold.

When I realized how much the United Kingdom weather dictated my life choices, it started to irritate me. It irritated me even more when someone told me that, living in Britain, "I had no choice but to accept the weather." Well, I chose not to accept it. I did something about it. Instead of spending my whole life moaning about it, like most people do where I am from, I used the skills I learned in my first business (my physio practice) to start my second business (my media business) and that gave me the *choice* of living in the much-warmer climate of Florida, all year round.

Within reason, I am free to live my life on my terms, unrestricted by the social norms and limits that are mostly passed on by someone who didn't figure out how to become exempt from them.

I believe that the quality of your life is dictated by the quality of the choices available to you. Being a successful business owner offers me and my family significantly better life choices. Life choices that my clinical skills could never afford me. I was a great clinician and although I enjoyed it, all that got me was a job working for a professional soccer team that pretty much dictated every aspect of my life from when I would work, what time I finished, how much I would earn, if I could have a day off, and right down to being told I had to answer my phone on vacation.

After quitting that job, my great clinical skills then landed me in a situation in my private practice where I was working 8 A.M. until 8 P.M., making lots of money, but still absent of the *choice* to be able to really do things and go places without worrying about taking a big hit financially if I didn't see patients. Clinical skills got me started but, in the end, severely limited the choices I could make in my life.

We all have options – but how many of us really have choices?

We all have the option to live in a nicer house – but how many really have the means? The concept of giving yourself "more choice" and having that as a goal is one of the most underestimated and overlooked things in life. The people chasing bigger houses and nicer cars, or some version of a "better lifestyle" (that they mostly can't define), haven't figured out that they don't really want either – they want the choice.

Write this down: *The people with the best lives have the best choices.* If you take nothing else from this book, it should be that. Wake up every day focusing on doing things that will expand the number of choices available to you and watch the quality of your life improve. Frustration is reduced, fulfilment is increased, and I guarantee you will even live a much simpler life.

My business success is primarily responsible for expanding the number of choices available to me, and my business success has happened because of my **business skills**. That is cause and effect. The cause – a dedication to learning and executing on business skills. The effect – an autonomous lifestyle. If you're looking for a reason to develop your business skills, you now have it: to give yourself more and better choices.

You show me a business owner *absent* of real business skills and I'll show you someone who, five years after starting his company, is still doing the things he was at the beginning. He's still "trapped," working every hour of the day and always justifying it by telling himself that it will be worth it "in the end."

You show me a business owner *absent* of business skills and I'll show a business owner who is always losing staff, or constantly short of cash when payroll comes around. That same business owner is the one always having to go back into the business to rescue it by working longer hours (limiting life choices) or paying wages out of his personal account (further limiting life choices). Business skills are the ultimate differentiator between business owners whose businesses are running *them* and business owners actually running *the company*.

Yet, and sadly, most business owners are not even 100 percent sure which skills they need to be successful – never mind how to polish them.

And that is the point of the second half of this book.

We're going to move on from the "general" leadership skills everyone needs to get through life (that can also serve you well in business) and look more closely at your role as the CEO of the private practice you started. We're going to get to the *business end of running a business* and look at the things you should be doing with your time if and when you finally step back from treating patients.

WHAT TO DO WITH TIME ONCE YOU'VE STOPPED TREATING PATIENTS

If you've already stopped treating patients, or you're about ready to jump off the cliff and do it, you'll know that one of the biggest issues you face is what to do with your time now that you have an empty schedule.

It's one of the biggest challenges clinicians face: what to do with the forty to fifty hours of time that you've got now that you've stepped back from patient care? (Spoiler: it's everything that we cover from here on out in the book.) It is also the one thing that defines the success of your practice from here on in. It's not just about what your employees do – it's actually as much about what *you* do.

You could argue that the two are interwoven. If you don't know what you're doing, then neither will your employees as one of your top jobs is to ensure that they know theirs. If you haven't prioritized this or you're not constantly communicating what you want from your team, then your company will struggle and flatline.

Every CEO has a set of major priorities that should consume their week. If you don't know what those priorities are, it is my intention that by the end of this book you will be able to look at your calendar and ask yourself on a Monday morning if what is on your calendar – and the time allocated to each task – reflects what a top CEO would be doing.

You'll be able to get more critical with where your time – the most important resource any CEO has available – is going and ask if it is appropriate to the needs of your company and its strategic objectives (which you set).

Understand it like this: stepping back from patient care is a huge decision for any practice owner. But what you do with your time is ultimately what determines how successful that decision will be – not that you did it.

If the first part of the book was important, this second part is vital for you as a business leader. It is where we take your ability to lead and bolt that on to the specific tasks that you are required to do as a CEO running a successful company. I'm going to give you the clarity you need about what your job as a CEO entails, what you should be doing in your day-to-day role, and how to get the skills and expertise needed to build a world-class private practice that grows and runs without you having to be involved with patients.

Are you ready?

THE THREE PHASES OF BUSINESS OWNERSHIP

We're going to start by looking at the different phases of business ownership. If there's confusion over what business owners actually do, there's also confusion over the definition of a business owner as well as what makes a "real business owner."

As far as I am concerned, anyone who is responsible for finding their own customers and paying their own taxes is a business owner. It's just that there are three different phases once a company has been created. I think it helps to understand those phases so you know how to move through them quickly and avoid getting stuck.

1. Self-Employed

You've likely heard the phrase "working *on* the business, not *in* the business." When you're self-employed, you're constantly working *in* the business. You're the one treating patients, you're the one who is answering the phone, you're cleaning the clinic, and you're updating the website as well as doing the social media.

When you are self-employed, your primary focus is on improving your craft. Every ounce of the value you're creating comes from your great clinical skills. You're full of energy and enthusiasm about your clinical skills and how you can use them to help people. It's a wonderful phase to be in. You're doing all of the things you enjoy about being a health care professional and you're often making a lot of money.

The best part? Most of the money you make is yours to keep.

There are very few, if any, employees and you feel like you're in control of most of what is happening. That feeling of being "in control" is also likely to be the primary reason you started the company in the first place. You love the feeling you get from driving to work and knowing you dictate your own schedule. You'll say that you started your business because you wanted "freedom," but what you really wanted was more control – or choice – over your day and more control over how you would provide a better service to your patients than you could at your last job (because you worked for a crappy boss or company who cared little about patients and was clueless about service.)

Back when I was in this self-employed phase, I recall that it was a time I had bundles of energy and enthusiasm for improving my clinical skills and my service. I wanted to get better and better with my treatment outcomes, and I wanted to make sure everything was perfect for the clients. That included everything from their treatment plans, how the clinic looked, the quality of the material that my business cards were printed on, right down to the T-shirts I wore to project the brand identity I wanted for myself. I wanted *everything* to be right. My thoughts were constantly consumed by these types of things back then.

All of these things are still important today. But back then, I made the mistake of thinking that if I just focused solely on these things, then I would make more money and more impact. And I did – but only to a certain point. And that point was reached about two years after starting my practice. I lost the enthusiasm and energy I had simply because I was overworked.

When you're self-employed, the prize for winning is you get to do everything.

You literally become a victim of your own success.

In the time since I've started working more closely with private practice owners, I see that many of them make the same mistake, and often in about the same time frame (usually about two years in). There's a lot of huff and puff but little in the way of strategic thinking or planning about how to get to the next phase.

What is more, if you pushed me on it, I'd say focusing solely on their "craft" (being a great clinician) is easily the number one mistake that keeps the self-employed physical therapist from ever creating a company of real and lasting value. That is value created beyond what the owner is able to provide themselves or on their own.

Why does this happen? It is very simple. The self-employed person struggles to give up control. They don't know how to get comfortable with being uncomfortable at the thought of someone else doing what they're good at.

Really, how could they? As I said earlier, that is often why they start the business in the first place. They start off doing everything and soon get very good at doing everything – but they're unable to recognize that having the ability to do everything perfectly is a curse, not a blessing.

If you're in this phase right now, the phrase to remember is, "I am really good at doing everything. The *problem* is I am really good at doing everything."

One of the best lessons I learned in the self-employed phase was to get comfortable with giving up control. In fact, *the* best lesson I learned was that growth and control work inversely. The more you want to grow, the more control you will need to give up. The more you will need to get comfortable with not being fully in control. It doesn't mean you won't be responsible or make the big decisions. It just means you need to learn the skill of determining which decisions you should be involved with and which ones you shouldn't. Prioritizing your time, your thoughts, and your energy will be one of the greatest skills you will ever learn.

From my experience, this is the spark that lights the flame to rapid business growth.

Whatever phase you're in, remember this as it will come in handy any time you're wrestling with not delegating tasks to your employees because you think you can do it better. As you will see on your CEO scorecard, delegation is one of the skills you absolutely must have to be able to run a successful private practice. I am sure you can do most things better – but the question is whether is it the best use of your time. If it isn't, and you're still going to do it, your business is going to get stuck. The skills you need to learn include outcome-based recruitment (see my best-selling book *The Physical Therapy Hiring Solution* for tips on how to do that), delegation, and holding people accountable to a clearly defined task. More on these things later.

2. Owner Operator

After being self-employed for a few years, and assuming you get fed up doing everything yourself, the next phase you will likely flow into is that of being an owner operator. This is where you likely get more staff, more patients (hopefully), a bigger office, cash flow gets tighter, and there's a need for a reliable marketing system to bring in revenue just to keep up with the higher expenses. Usually, all this happens at the same time as trying to treat the twenty to twenty-five patients a week who got you started in the first place.

In this phase, you start to employ other people to do things for you, although each time you do, you're not always exactly sure why you did. Payroll goes up – but you've still got less time on your hands.

In my humble opinion, this is the worst phase to be in as a business owner simply because you're never ready to deal with all of the variables and challenges thrown at you. It's also the one where most people get stuck.

Congratulations! Your great clinical skills have landed you with a whole new set of new problems that no college lecturer ever prepared you for. You're about to start getting tested before you've even had the lesson.

I'd describe this phase as being stuck in quicksand. No matter how hard you work or how hard you try, you can never make any real, sustainable progress. At best you feel like the only thing you're doing is keeping your head above water. There's little, if any, sustainable progress – you're only ever balancing the equilibrium.

Being an owner operator is also a bit like *Groundhog Day*. Like the movie of the same name, you're literally reliving the same events of yesterday, day after day. And that would be fine if good, positive things were happening. But each day usually involves a series of unwelcome or tedious problems recurring in the exact same way.

For example, it could be the bills that were sent out with the wrong codes (again), the staff constantly quitting, the staff constantly not showing up, or the staff showing up, but showing up late or always bringing high drama.

It could be the marketing not working, or not being done at all, or perhaps a repeat complaint caused by the same process not being followed by the same employee. Of course, the person responsible will tell you it's never their fault and that the process is flawed, so off you go again to rewrite it for the thirteenth time. And so the cycle goes on and on. Mind-numbing challenges and tedious issues keep cropping up, but because you're too busy treating patients, you never get time to get your head above water and fix them. The predicament that your business is in causes you to constantly get distracted from fixing what is needed. Instead of making progress, you're constantly fighting fires. The only problem is you're too busy putting them out to ever notice who is starting them.

What is the predicament?

You are starved of time.

Your inability to give up control (that you carried over from the self-employed phase) has forced you to continue to think that you can do everything yourself.

And, of course, you can.

You're world class at getting the stuff done that needs to be done urgently. There's nothing *important* in your business anymore – it's all *urgent*. And you're good at meeting urgent deadlines. If only there were forty-eight hours in one day and two of you. Wouldn't your clinic would be ten times as big as it is today?

Seriously, most owner operators find themselves in this exact situation for years – constantly reacting to things that are not being done, or being done incorrectly.

At best, even if things are being done, you're spending your whole week paranoid just in case something isn't. Your thoughts are consumed by everything except how to fix the problem at its root source or grow the business past today's crisis.

In this phase, most people are so consumed by the trivial many that they can't spot the important few. They wouldn't recognize a problem-solving idea if it was delivered in the mail in a bright red box with a gold ribbon on top. It's safe to say that the operator is not running the business – they are being run *by* it. And there's definitely a few questions about why this business was started in the first place.

Sound familiar?

If it does, here's where it goes really wrong.

When you enter this type of cycle, you're possibly so desperate to get out if it that you'll try literally anything that comes along that promises to solve the problem quickly for you. The only problem is that when you go down that route, it usually creates more problems because you were trying to solve the wrong problem in the first place.

You might have had the right answer – but the question was wrong.

You fixed the hamstring, but the problem was in the lower back.

In this phase, you're being pulled apart by the obligations you think you have to fulfil. You're treating your loyal patients and still trying to do the work required of an owner. There's little, if any, satisfaction or progress in either area.

STOP SERVING THE BEER AND PRETZELS

Bizarrely, some owner operators even justify staying in the seat of operator because they think they'll have "more control" if they do. They tell themselves that if they stay in the treatment room all day – treating as many patients as is possible – then they are able to run the business better.

Really? How is that even remotely possible?

That by spending forty hours per week in the treatment room, you can run a better business? That is like the pilot of a Boeing 747 thinking the best thing he can do is to leave the cockpit and serve the beer and pretzels to the passengers while the plane flies across the ocean unattended.

Candidly, most private practice owners are doing just this. They're guilty of serving beer and pretzels to their patients when what they should be doing is sitting in the cockpit and flying the plane. They should know that the passengers are getting their drinks and refreshments, but they should find out by checking in with the senior flight attendant, whom they hired to make sure the passengers are happy. This means they can stay focused on monitoring the flight plan and the weather up ahead and ensuring all of the vital dials in the cockpit are showing as they should be to ensure a smooth and safe flight that lands at the correct destination.

The lesson to learn quickly in this phase is that you've likely grown the business without developing the structure.

Every decision up to this point was made on impulse or on what appeared to solve the day's problem. And you made impulsive decisions simply because you're out of time. You're out of time because you failed at prioritizing. You prioritized treating patients – serving beer and pretzels – over leading your business and doing the work that is required at the business end of the business.

3. The CEO

By contrast, when you get to the CEO level, you're constantly and only working "on" the business (and "on" yourself.) That means your focus is on adding and creating sustainable value that goes beyond what you alone can provide. If there's a fire, you don't rush to put it out. Your team puts it out and you figure out who or what started it and then build a better process to make sure it doesn't happen again.

Everything you are doing or committing time to is designed to find more time for you in the long run. You're obsessed with leverage. If you're committing forty hours to something, it should be a repeatable process that you won't have to get involved in anymore.

You're starting to work smart, not just hard.

As a CEO, you're getting clever with how you think, how you make decisions, and who you hire. You realize that most of the problems you had in the beginning where "who" problems – not just "how" problems – and you understand the importance of leveraging other people's time (and possibly someone else's money) to get more things done than you ever could on your own.

Your focus is now on building a team, company structure, creating repeatable systems, and leading and coaching other people to be better. You've learned to be okay with giving up control. You're comfortable with the idea that other people can do tasks – even if not as well as you.

You realize that five people doing things at 80 percent of your standard adds up to a total sum of value that is a lot more than you could achieve on your own – even if you do it better. The company success happens because it is the sum of all its parts and it's stronger than any one individual.

You're developing your culture, you're spending more time on recruitment, and you've implemented a cash flow forecast as well as the dashboards that tell you where your team's performance has dropped (so you can coach it back up). You're able to do all of this because you have time – you're not in the treatment room looking after patients most of the day. You're doing the job needed of you by your business.

As the CEO, you're running the company instead of the company running you.

This is easily the most enjoyable phase to be in and usually the most lucrative in terms of time and money. The reward certainly justifies the means at this level and that happens because you're focusing more on creating the machine that is your business – on designing it – than actually being trapped in it.

As the CEO of the business, you are responsible for specific things such as finance, accounting, operations, marketing, sales, hiring, firing, training, and development, to name just a few – and you're always thinking about them simultaneously. But you now have time to do so because you're not thinking about Mrs. Smith and exercises for her spondylosis.

You've moved on from thinking about your Mulligan or McKenzie techniques and instead you're obsessing over things like:

- Creating a budget or a strategic growth plan

- Analyzing numbers (and turning them into activity so that you can work out what needs to change)
- Creating a marketing plan that addresses who your perfect patient is, what message will resonate with that patient, and what media you're most likely to reach them on
- How you attract and retain A players
- Creating a culture that inspires growth and where outcomes and results are more important than people working hard and being friends
- Evaluating risks and considering the second-order consequence of all your decisions

These are the things that are now consuming your thoughts. On top of that, you're developing and honing the skills of delegation and prioritization so that the right things get done by the right people. When you crack this nut, your business will soar.

Ultimately, and in the end, all of the success that you have or do not have comes down to one thing: how well you can prioritize your three major resources (time, money, and people). The business owner who is winning knows how to prioritize. The one who is losing hasn't figured out how to diagnose the real problem in their business and is therefore prioritizing the allocation of resources incorrectly. Working hard on the wrong things.

Over the next few chapters, we're going to take a closer look at some of the actions that will help you get better at allocating and prioritizing your resources. They include:

1. Setting the vision: creating the growth plan/roadmap
2. Managing the cash: achieving financial clarity
3. Find the A players: recruiting the right people
4. Managing the A players: creating the right culture
5. Constantly honing your skills

At this point, and before we move to the next chapter, you'll need your CEO job description and scorecard handy. Be sure to download it from here: **www.paulgough.com/leadership-resource**

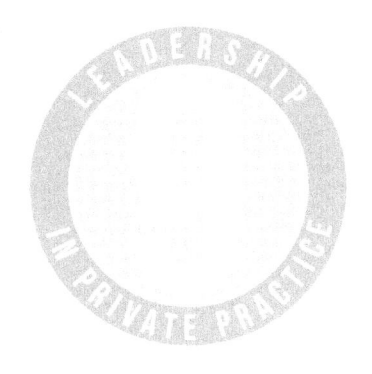

CREATE THE GROWTH PLAN

To drive your business forward, to make real and lasting progress, it's vital to know where you are actually going. It's elementary to suggest that you need to know what the target is before you can hit it. But I have to ask: do you *really* know *what* you want? Just as important, do you know *how* you will actually achieve it?

There's no shortage of business owners who can tell you what they want. In fact, most could tell you in an instant. They'll usually say something arbitrary like, "The plan is to make $1,000,000" or "The plan is to build a chain of five clinics that I can sell for $5,000,000."

Here's the mistake they all make. What they describe here is not the plan – it is the outcome. They're telling you what they want. And like I just said, they nearly all know what they want. But what they lack is a road map – a plan – to get them there. Very few business owners can ever describe what the road to Oz looks like. Hence, very few ever make it to see the Wizard.

And by the way – you'll hear people around you say the same type of thing all the time. "The plan is to buy a bigger house" or "the plan is to get a new job next year." No. That is the outcome. You need a plan to get both of those things. Coincidentally, the people who talk like this are also the ones who are perpetually lost in their lives. They're full of great intentions – but their goals rarely ever materialize. They have no growth plan.

Your growth plan is essentially your road map to reaching your growth targets and is the first and most important step in growing your business from where it is today to where you want it to be. Crucially, it also helps you reach those targets in your desired time frame. A successful growth plan clearly outlines your objectives and the steps and activities you need to implement, in a given time frame, to achieve these objectives. Essentially, you are documenting your long-term vision and strategic goals.

Creating a growth plan is a vital task for a CEO. Everything that happens in your business must be about taking you toward the goal or target you've set – in the time frame you set. Whether you call it your vision, your goal, your target on the wall, your outcome, or something else, it is simply the description of what you want to achieve from your business. Why you're in it in the first place.

But here's the point you must grasp: the growth plan isn't just about naming your target. No. It's about infusing the *what* with the *how*.

If the *what* is the ultimate goal – "the $1,000,000 pay day within five years" – then the *how* is the road map. It lays out the path that you're going to have to walk and the milestones you'll have to pass to reach your outcome.

Think about Google Maps. It's a very successful application. It does the job of telling you exactly how to get to where you want to be. It doesn't take you there – it shows you how to get there. It provides the route. In fact, it usually offers more than one route and you get to decide which one you will take. One is faster, one is more scenic, and one is perhaps is free of tolls. It populates three different paths and then you decide which route you want to take.

Why does it work? How does it provide the accurate route map? Simple. You are able to input the final destination or end goal. You are able to describe exactly where you want to go. If it knows where you are now, and you tell it where you want to go, it will produce a clear road map for you to follow. Best of all, it will even allow you to follow the route so you can look for indicators or markers on the journey that tell you if you're on or off course. These are like milestones to keep you on track that should also be part of your business growth plan.

What is more, it even tells you how long it should take to get there.

If you're going slower than you should be, the time frame expands. If you're going faster, the time frame reduces. There are a lot of similarities between Google Maps and your business growth plan. The most important thing to remember, though, is that the growth plan doesn't achieve the outcome for you – it simply tells you what to do and when.

You document the goal or target and then create a series of milestones that let you know if you're on track. Against every milestone is an agreed-upon standard that lets the business know if they're on track to achieving the bigger growth goal.

For example, you want to achieve a $500,000 revenue business and you conclude that you will need 50 new patients per month to do it. The *what* you want to achieve is the $500,000. *How* you will achieve it is by hitting the 50 new patients per month milestone. When you know the mini milestones, it allows you to orchestrate your team's focus and prioritize their time correctly. Your weekly marketing meeting takes on a completely

GET YOUR FREE RESOURCE KIT: PAULGOUGH.COM/LEADERSHIP-RESOURCE

different level of intensity and focus when you know that you're currently coming up short to the tune of 20 patients per month.

If you know after the first two weeks of January that you're only at five new patients, then you know that you must change something. The road map is telling you that the milestones are not being passed. As the CEO, you then get the chance to do your job and prioritize the time and money that your team is spending on marketing to improve results and make up the shortfall before the year is over. You get to look at the results and change the activities in real time instead of waiting for your accountant to tell you that you missed the cut – again.

The typical business owner will tell you he wants to reach an outcome – often a monetary figure that gets higher every year (usually to compensate for failed previous years) – and he'll set about trying to achieve it. There's no shortage of hard work or sweat equity put into the business. But there's a consistent theme that emerges. Despite working harder, the business owner never seems to hit the target.

Despite popular wisdom, and as many are finding out, working hard and hitting targets do not always go hand in hand. Hustle is fine as long as you are hustling down the right path.

It's been my experience that working hard while following a detailed plan often does result in hitting targets. That is the value of the growth plan. But remember, just because you create it, that doesn't mean you will automatically achieve your target. The CEO's job is to use it as a tool that guides you and your thinking so you can change your actions if you find yourself off course.

So, what specifically is in your growth plan? Make sure you're considering the following components. (There's a downloadable template of this growth plan available at www.paulgough.com/leadership-resource.)

1. What's The Strategic Intent?

This is your attempt to verbalize what you want to achieve. What will be the end result of the blood, sweat, and tears you're giving to your business? Your strategic intent could be, "To scale to a four-location private practice that does not deal with insurance companies and within five years allows you to own the buildings your clinics are housed in." It could be, "To grow to a national chain of 50 clinics with one clinic in every state in the country in the next ten years." You're not saying *how* you will do it, you're just saying *what* will be the result and *when* you will have done it.

It's a high-level, 35,000-foot view of what you're wanting to achieve and by when. And it's important that you constantly remind yourself of that view. I carry my growth plan everywhere I go. It's always in my bag so that whenever I am on a plane, on a train, a long Uber journey, or during times in my office when I am feeling lost, I can quickly and easily go back to it. I find it pulls me back up the strategic level at which I need to be.

When you're running a business, it is so easy to get sucked into the weeds or the minutiae and before you know it you're stuck there. The devil might be in the details – but it's also a place that a lot of business owners have trouble escaping.

Personally, I like to leave the details to the people I recruited because of their detail-oriented skills. I will freely admit I am not a detail person. Sure, I will spot things and I will notice things, but I am not the one doing the inspecting. I employ people to do that so I can remain creative and free to think about the strategies required to grow my business – to drive my business. It is the perfect arrangement.

As you consider your recruitment, you have to think about these things and know precisely what you, as the CEO, should and shouldn't be getting involved in.

As we discussed in chapter 2, when you do too much of what I call "tactical" or "detail" work, your business inevitably grinds to a halt. Any business owner who is constantly fixing things, doing "busy" work, or always fighting fires is caught up in the tactics. This often goes hand in hand with a business that has stopped growing despite the owner working harder.

So, what's the difference between tactics and strategy? Simple. Tactics are the means to achieving the overall bigger picture – the strategy.

You need to be the one coming up with the strategy.

If you've hired the right people, it's also your job to let them get on with executing that strategy for you. They've been employed to take care of the detail. It's important that you're not afraid to get involved in the tactics or dive into the weeds to fix things, but it's equally important that you're not spending all your time there. The absolute bare minimum ratio to shoot for is eighty-twenty. That is, 20 percent of your week is spent thinking about the strategies of your business and 80 percent is spent actually executing them (tactics).

The business owners who are energized are the ones who are working at the strategic level of their business. They're doing the "thinking" and mostly working *on* the business.

Most owners who are struggling or feel stuck are in that position because they're spending time on tactics that aren't driven by strategy.

Ask yourself how you feel about your business at any given time and I bet you'll find some truth in what I've just explained. When you're energized, you're strategic. When you're drained of energy, you've been dragged back into the weeds. This is a great way of recognizing when you must shift gears and get back to the perch the CEO should sit on, looking down on the business.

THE "10-80-10" PRINCIPLE OF LEADERSHIP

Let me give you a couple of examples of tactical versus strategic work.

Fixing the sales script is tactical. Fixing the marketing message and ensuring that the person using the script has been hired and trained properly is strategic.

Spending time on your clinic's logo or company branding is tactical. Considering the marketing message or the unique selling proposition (USP) that is on each of these things and explaining what the company stands for is strategic.

In hiring, doing the actual interview and asking the questions is tactical. Considering who you want to hire, what problem they will solve, and what skills they will need as well as how they fit into the company org chart is strategic.

In all three of these examples, there is one thing in common: you're spending time thinking. What you realize as a CEO is that sometimes it doesn't feel like you're doing any actual work. You're mostly thinking and coaching. If you're doing it right, you'll have a pen in your hand or be standing next to a white board, mapping everything out for your people to execute on.

Strategy governs tactical execution. Sadly, most business owners never get to this level and yet it's where you really step into your own as a business owner. I've spent as little as 60 minutes on some of the best marketing campaigns I've ever put together. Those campaigns then required a month of tactical implementation by my team. I checked it off at the end. In doing so, I executed on what I call the 10-80-10 principle I use to get things done.

As the CEO, I get involved in the first 10 percent of the project as I explain what I want and make sure everyone has the resources they need and knows the time frame in which I want this done. The team then goes off and does the tactical work required of bringing the project to life (80 percent). Then I get involved again at the end to make sure my plan has come to fruition (10 percent).

I must get involved at the end. Otherwise, I am abdicating and, as we discussed earlier, that is not what great leaders do.

I can do the same with hiring. The strategic level requires me to think about the qualities we're looking for – the tasks that, if achieved, will make this person successful as well as what skills we need. I can do that in a white board session in an hour (10 percent) and yet it could take my team up to eight weeks in the recruitment process to find the person I want to spend my time on during an interview (80 percent). I often still make the final hiring decision, but it only takes a couple of hours to do so (10 percent).

The entire process was created to protect my time, leverage the time of the team, and utilize my best skills as the CEO. It works for three different businesses in two different countries. As I always say, business is business. The skills required in the UK are no different from the USA. The skills required in running a media business are no different from those of a private practice. Only people who are struggling will try to tell you that the circumstances of their business are somehow "different" or that the rules of business success do not apply to them (they mostly don't know the rules, but that's a different story altogether).

Tactics are very important – the choice of the job site, the questions we ask at interview, etc., but not nearly as important as the overall strategy. That's about considering the outcomes for the role, the specific skills required, and the previous job roles and values of the person that we want.

Getting to a point where you're thinking more strategically takes time. It's a skill you have to hone. But when you nail it, it means you're not going to be involved in the day-to-day running of the business as much. In that way, you've freed up your time to continue to make improvements in and grow the business. You can think more about your company structure and the people you need to get to the next level – should you wish to go there.

If you stay at the tactical level, you will remain stuck. You'll always feel like you're "spinning your wheels." There's activity – but very little accomplishment.

To conclude, strategy is vital. Becoming more strategic in your thinking will coincide with more and faster progress in your business. If you want that, it's a wonderful choice to be able to exercise.

2. Consider Your Core Client (Perfect Patient)

As part of any plan for growth, you must also consider your core client. You need clients and patients to grow a private practice, but it's not just the volume of them that determines how successful you will be. No, before you decide *how many* of them you want, you first decide *who* you want.

If you market to a patient who doesn't really value their health enough to want to pay for it – which might be true of younger people with less disposable income – then you will need a lot more of those patients calling you as they'll not spend as much money as, say, a lady in her sixties who does value her health and is willing to spend money to feel better. There's another example of strategic thinking that will save you time and make you money.

To easily figure out who your perfect patient really is, just answer this question: "Who spends the most money with you with the least effort?" Who is the person who loves to buy from you and does so without resistance? There is a person in your office who can't wait for any excuse to pop up to spend money with you – what does that person look like?

It never ceases to amaze me how many business owners ignore this question in pursuit of patients who are harder to find, harder to work with, or who they "enjoy" working with because they have some affinity to the field they are in (such as CrossFit or soccer).

Business is hard enough at the best of times. There's no need to make it harder.

When you get crystal clear on who your perfect patient is, it also allows you to evolve the company with that person firmly in mind. Your hiring decisions, your customer service experience, your marketing message, your upsells, and your client testimonials can all be made more relevant and more impactful. The compound effect of understanding who your perfect patient is and implanting decisions with that person in mind is stunning.

You might not think you have such a "perfect patient" in your practice, but you do.

Within every private practice, it is a mathematical fact that someone spends the most money with you. Even if you only have 25 patients in your database, this is still true. Some type of patient with some type of ailment is spending more with you than the others. I am not saying don't treat the others, I am saying make it your strategic intent to go actively looking for more of your most desirable patient.

Figure out who is spending the money and then build your entire business and broader marketing plan around finding more of that type of person.

It *could* be a female in her sixties who comes to see you with lower back pain. Or it *could* be a guy in his thirties who likes to go to CrossFit. From this far, I don't know. But I know for sure that this person already exists in your business and it's vital you root him or her out. As a CEO, that is your job and it requires a dedication to understanding the principles of successful marketing. Everything becomes more difficult if you don't do this – especially when you try to scale or spend money on marketing (for help, get my best-selling book on marketing, *New Patient Accelerator Method*, from www.paulgoughbooks.com).

It's very rare that you'll find a successful small business where the CEO doesn't have serious input in the clinic's marketing. Do not abdicate this responsibility. I am all for the CEO having a marketing assistant who is doing the tactics – even outsourcing to marketing agencies who have more expertise in the tactical work of Google Ads etc, – but as the CEO of a small private practice, you must be driving the marketing at the strategic level.

As part of your annual growth plan, you're considering (and reconsidering) if the perfect patient is still the perfect patient – or have there been any changes? Are you seeing a new type of perfect patient evolve who comes into your clinic, is a pleasure to work with, agrees to the treatment they need, and is happy to pay at a level that allows you provide the service they desire?

3. Primary Objective (Target on the Wall)

This is getting laser focused on what success looks like. It's about writing things down and getting clear on a specific target that must be achieved in a specific period of time. It can't be vague. You can't just say you want to "grow your business" – you have to say by how much and by when.

It could be that within three years you want to reach $500,000 in total revenue with a healthy 20 percent profit margin that includes a $75,000 fair market salary paid to you.

That is specific, measurable, attainable, and time bound. There can be no arguments about whether or not you achieved your primary objective.

You either did or you didn't.

You're either on the way or you're lost and have some serious ground to make up.

4. SWOT Analysis

A SWOT analysis is an exercise that you do with your team to consider the strengths, weaknesses, opportunities, and threats to your company. Let's take a look at some examples.

Strengths: this might be your marketing power, your great customer service, or a huge past patient database that you can market to at will.

Weaknesses: this might be a lack of a senior leadership team, or that you're running on fumes with little cash on hand to fuel faster growth.

Opportunities: these could include partnering with health professionals in the area or to add new marketing streams such as community events or digital media

Threats: threats could include being unable to find good clinical staff in the required time frame or the fact you have a single point of failure in one great employee who would leave the business exposed if she left.

When you have considered and then documented all of these factors, it allows you to consider what action or resources you must allocate to develop your strengths, reduce the risk of your weaknesses, mitigate the threats, and maximize the opportunities. This is a strategic exercise and it could be done every three months. That is because opportunities evolve, strengths get fragile, and weaknesses can easily get weaker.

Really, most of the value of this exercise is in everyone getting out of the practice.

It's hard to spot an opportunity when you're constantly treating patients or thinking about how to get more followers on social media (both of which are tactical). What is more, this exercise has extra value simply because you are bringing your team together. It gives your team an opportunity to have their say and offer an input into how the business will achieve its goals.

One thing that you will never give up as the CEO is the *what* you want to achieve, but you're definitely going to have to allow your team some kind of ownership over *how* it is achieved. A SWOT analysis is the perfect opportunity to do this.

I've learned that the more that you do things like this, that involve your team and their ideas, the more you reduce the input and day-to-day direction that you need to provide. You are breeding independence from you and your direction. This frees up more of your most valuable resource – time.

As you will no doubt pick up on as you read this book, the spark in your business growth happens when you and your time are optimized.

And that only happens when you become world class and prioritize tasks that are designed to free up time to allow you to think more critically. Thinking critically allows you to spot different opportunities and solutions to challenges.

I'm as serious as I can be when I tell you that every single thing you're doing should be about freeing you up so that you can remain creative and able to think critically and strategically about your business. That is where all of your value as the CEO of the company comes from. You have to get there ASAP.

5. Key Strategies

Your key strategies are the things that will guide your business toward the overall target you outlined earlier. The key strategies act as a guardrail for you, the CEO, to make sure your team isn't swerving off the road. If you are, how can you expect to get where you want to go? You might have left Kansas, but the goal is to get to see the Wizard in Oz.

Identifying your target is one thing, but the thing that will take you there is identifying the key strategies – and then working on them. The key words are "working on them." It is one thing to identify them, but if you don't work on them – actually see them through – then this is a spectacular failure of leadership.

Great CEOs don't construct ten rickety bridges that are only half built. Instead, they commit to building four steel walkways that are finished and get everyone safely to the other side.

If you've been in business for any length of time, think of all of the time you've ever wasted in developing a plan that isn't shaping up; in sitting down with your team and telling them what you want to achieve only to find that yet again you all get distracted by the trivial issues that crop up each day.

When this happens, chances are, you allowed the team to slip back into doing work that *they* deemed urgent – but that keeps the business stuck.

I've come to realize that, given the choice, staff always seem to default to work that is instantly gratifying and keeps away the wolf from the door – rather than favoring work that makes the wolf irrelevant. It's only natural. They don't want you to get hurt and they don't really understand what drives business growth. It is your job to spell this out over and over again. You'll never be able to do anything more valuable for your company than overcommunicate the key strategies that you want them to work on – and why. Always communicate the why. Without the why, you don't get to the what or the how. You just stay stuck in drama.

Here's what I want you to grasp: In the end, you will realize that almost nothing is *really* that urgent. The only thing that is truly urgent is the work that is required to stop feeling like you had to do urgent work in the first place. When you adopt that mind-set, you're on your way to rapid growth.

So, what are examples of key strategies? Check out the following examples that I've plucked from previous strategy meetings with my own team:

1. Leverage relationships with local healthcare professionals to ensure a consistent and reliable stream of new patients.
2. Develop an online/digital presence to reach tens of thousands more potential clients that take us beyond relying on referrals from past patients or insurance companies.
3. Develop an in-house staff training program that improves both the clinical and customer care experience.
4. Find and recruit a marketing manager to ensure that our plan to recruit 80 new patients per month is successfully executed.
5. Create scorecards and ensure that all staff understand the outcomes of their roles.
6. Implement daily, weekly, and monthly reporting (including dashboards and performance reviews) that improve individual and overall team results.
7. Develop our leadership bench, including structure and rhythm of team meetings.

These seven strategies are examples that would guide all of the tactical decisions you'd make in a given period of time – say, a year. They would allow you to create a series of ten to twelve tasks underneath each strategy and then appoint someone in your team to be responsible – to be held accountable – for seeing that specific strategy through to completion.

What you might find interesting is that as the years have gone on, and to allow my group of businesses to continue to grow, I start any team discussion about key strategies with the phrase, "Remember, whatever we're about to agree on, it can't include me being responsible for its completion."

I am basically telling my team that whatever we need to do, it needs to happen without "PG" marked as responsible for it happening (we always add the initials of the team member who is responsible for that strategy). If I didn't do this, I would find myself with five amazing strategies – the only problem being that I would be the bottleneck in all of them.

In the beginning, you'll want to be involved in some of them, but as you progress, and if you've recruited well, you'll want to adopt the position of overseeing the execution of the strategies – making sure they get done – instead of doing them all yourself. It's a fine line to cross, but when you get there, you'll know you're running a business and, at last, it's not running you.

Some key things to understand about developing key strategies: these key strategies are like levers that, when pulled, make a huge impact and take you closer to bigger objectives. They are markers for you to always be able to check your activity against your accomplishment. It is easy to get sucked into tactical work, but if you do, your business will remain at the level it's at right now. Fine, if that's what you want. But for most, it isn't. If you're not working on the key strategies, you're doing busy work and your business is about to become inefficient. You'll work hard – but all you will get is tired. You will have allowed the trivial many to get in the way of the important few.

6. Financials: Past, Current, and Projections

As part of your growth plan, you must consider some aspect of your business's financial data. At the very least, that should include facts about your past performance. Take a look at your total revenue over the past three to five years and see how it trended from year to year. The trend is your friend. It gives you clues about what the future could hold. Once you consider all of that, you can then set about creating projections for the year ahead.

Of course, the past isn't always a good indicator of how the future will go, but in the case of business, it is more reliable than anything else. Why? Well, many business owners are making the same decisions today that they did five years ago – in that respect, the future is already known. It's going to be exactly how it has been in the past.

Simply put, if you want to know why your business (or your life) looks the way it does today, look at the decisions you made in the past. If you want to know how it will look in the future, inspect the decisions you're making today.

When you look at the previous and most recent years' results for your company, it is much easier to look at and sensibly consider realistic future financial targets.

This is much better and likely to be way more accurate than simply looking at what you wanted last year and then adding 20 percent in the hopes that things will change just because you're due a streak of good luck.

Financial clarity is vital for a successful CEO. So much so that there's a full chapter coming up on the importance of your financial clarity (and perhaps, someday soon, an entire book?).

7. Critical Drivers (Displayed via Dashboards)

Your critical drivers are the indicators – milestones – that tell you how well you're doing against the road map you've created. If you're driving from Washington to New York, and you're heading in the right direction, you'll know it before you get there because you'll have passed important buildings or landmarks on your approach.

Remember the days before GPS? We used to have to pull over and ask someone how to get to where we wanted to go. "If you see a set of new houses, you're going in the wrong direction. However, if you see a school on your left, you're on the right track." Anyone else remember hearing things like that?

The person we asked was giving us the milestones to check off to make sure we were heading in the right direction. It's how we all found our way in the olden days (before Google Maps), and the premise is still true today for business owners like you and me: if you keep an eye on the milestones, you'll know you're on the path that will lead to your destination.

Critical – or success – drivers offer the same reassurance or guidance for a business owner as a traveller looking for directions in a foreign country. They're simply performance indicators – success or failure – that tell you ahead of time how you're doing.

The reason I love critical drivers is because if you monitor your business's critical drivers, then you'll always know if you're going to hit – or miss – your target. Even better, you'll know it ahead of time. If you monitor your diet and exercise, you won't need to get on the scales every week as you'll already know what you're going to weigh.

Likewise, you won't need the report card from the accountant or your bookkeeper to tell you how well you're doing. Not if you already know that your number of leads was down 50 percent or your average patient spend was $250 less than it should be. These are just two examples of critical drivers that you should have displayed in a dashboard that tell you what you're likely to make at the end of the month or year. Other critical drivers could include things like your arrival rate or your phone conversion rate.

In my clinic, and across all of my business – in both countries – we affectionately call this dashboard our "cockpit." Every pilot steps into his or her cockpit and has a series of dials that reveal the health of the plane in real time. I need the same for my business in order for it to land at its destination safely, and on time.

The best thing about dashboards is they allow you to turn numbers into information that reveals clues about your business and who is doing – or perhaps *not* doing – well in your company.

Every top CEO lives by dashboards that allow them to connect the numbers they're seeing to the activities of their people. If you monitor and measure activity, you can change it appropriately by allocating resources or doing a better job of prioritizing. Do that and your results will change. Don't do that and you'll always get what you've always been getting.

If you create a financial plan that has an outcome attached – the target on the wall or primary objective – then the critical drivers become the *standards* that are required of your team. When these standards are met, they give you a very good shot at hitting your target. And, like I've discussed earlier in this book, raising your standard is the key to raising the performance of your business.

I'll discuss more on this in the chapter on financial clarity, but it's safe to say that understanding the importance of critical drivers and then checking them against our required standard on a weekly basis was a true game changer for the Paul Gough group of companies worldwide.

8. Marketing Requirements

A well-developed marketing plan is one of the greatest tools in the tool belt of a top CEO. It runs parallel to any annual budget and shows you exactly who needs to do what, how much you have to spend, and what specific results you need from any of the marketing channels on which you choose to spend your time and money.

The marketing plan considers the budget (how much you will spend), the cost of getting new patients, the marketing message, the frequency of ads, and even what to do if the ads don't work.

I budget at least one full day to create a comprehensive marketing plan for each of my businesses, then we review them each month and quarter.

The first time that you do it, it might take longer. However, each year you do it, you're refining it and it gets easier and more accurate as your predictions start coming more from fact and experience rather than hope.

9. Staffing

The best time to hire people is in preparation for needing them. By the time you need them, it's often too late – you've likely got chaos happening. That's why you should consider staffing as a vital part of your growth plan.

If your plan is a set of projections – major assumptions – about how your business is going to grow, then with that comes the knowledge that meeting your goal will (more often than not) involve adding people.

Here's why: if you're saying that you're going to grow by 50 percent, but you're not adding additional people to the team to help you do it or deal with it, you might be underestimating the situation. Or, more candidly, you're just delusional. You can decide. But either way, you're not living in the real world of business growth.

If you're about to jump from 50 new patients per month to 100 because your annual target has doubles, then how will you answer the phone and talk to all those extra people? How will you service them? How will you deliver on the promise your marketing is making? How will you maintain the customer service standards that your patients have come to expect?

Every increase in patient volume will bring its own additional stresses to your staffing capacity so it pays to be critical (and realistic) with your thinking about how your growth will require more staff.

Of course, there is the scenario in which you're not planning to add any more patients and you're going to grow your bottom line by doubling your prices (my favorite way to grow profits!).

And if that's your plan, you might not need more staff.

But then again, you still might.

If you're doubling prices, you might need to double your standards of customer care or the time you're spending on the phone helping patients see the value of the new price. If so, you'll still need more people. Either way, the fact you're thinking about it ahead of time significantly increases the likelihood that you will get it right.

I've learned the hard way that hiring is always best done when you're planning for success rather than reacting to success. When I hold CEO Mastermind meetings with clinic owners who want to talk about potential future hires, I know they've got a handle on their business. The ones who constantly tell me they need to replace people who recently quit, or needed to be chucked off the bus (a polite way of saying "fired"), then I know there's a little bit of drama going on in that practice. There's a need for more of the owners' focus to be placed on recruitment on subsequently developing the scorecards of new recruits.

Okay, so those are just some of the things you would need to consider when doing your growth plan. Suffice it to say that it is vital that you take the time to do it.

It doesn't need to be *War and Peace* or even the length of *Fifty Shades of Grey*. It is a document you will create in two days the first time and then revise annually.

Once you've done it, as I said earlier, carry it with you everywhere. It serves as a guide for reminding you of the most important considerations in your business – how you should prioritize and allocate your resources so that you can hit your goals in the most efficient way possible.

If I was to sum up your growth plan in true 80/20 fashion (where 20 percent of the activities produce 80 percent of the results), I'd tell you that getting the key strategies right and recruiting the right people to help you execute those strategies is going to be what makes or breaks your business success. The question is, will you make the time to do this?

All right, on to the next chapter. In this one, we're going to look at every business owner's favorite topic – finance! (Just kidding.) We are going to look at it, but I know it's most practice owners' biggest nightmare. Looking at finance reports is like eating sludge to most (my younger self included). It's the Kryptonite to their amazing clinical skills. If anything is going to derail a fast-growing private practice, it's a lack of financial clarity or savviness. That's why this next chapter is so important to you.

Let's be blunt for a moment. The reality is that, for most business owners, finance is an afterthought. They never expected to actually make any money and by the time they are, they're now too busy to create a finance department or get any real clarity surrounding their money.

And yet, it's likely to be the thing that determines whether or not you grow past where you are now and, most importantly, if you do it profitably.

Ready to look at what is involved in getting financial clarity? Turn the page and let's look together.

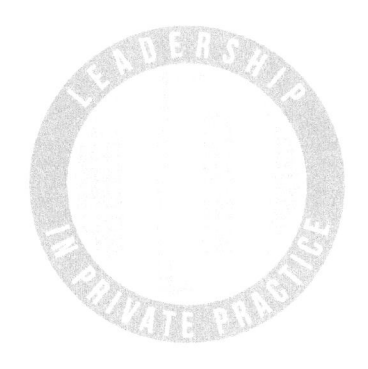

UNDERSTANDING THE NUMBERS AND DEVELOPING FINANCIAL CLARITY

Once you've created the growth plan, you need to be as accurately informed as possible about your progress. This is why you need financial clarity. Top CEOs don't just know their numbers – they know what the numbers mean and, most importantly, what to do to change the numbers if they don't read well. There's a difference.

It's true that most clinic owners hate looking at their numbers.

They'll say they're "not good at numbers," but what they're really saying is they just don't like to look at the ones they're seeing.

It's usually because their business is performing so poorly that they don't want to look at them and yet, ironically, the ones who would benefit from knowing their numbers are the ones who seem to shy away from looking at them.

The ones who are doing well – and know their numbers – seem to want to know even more. There's a pattern there, and it doesn't take a genius to work out what it is. The ones who know their numbers – who could arguably *not* look at their numbers every week – are the ones who are having success. In case it is missed, they're having success *because* they're looking.

The ones who are not looking are missing success because they don't know their numbers and therefore don't know what to do to improve them. If you don't know what's going wrong – how can you realistically expect to change it?

A tired business owner is the sign of one who doesn't really understand the numbers. There's profit missing from the business that they expected – and their only response is to shout at someone to work harder or do better. They're not sure on what, they just think that if the tone is more aggressive or their voice is louder, then things will change.

But they never do.

It's madness, but it's so often the case that this is the "norm."

It may be the norm amongst *un*successful business owners – but I can tell you it's far from the truth for the ones who are so successful that you'd want to swap places with them.

Sadly, most clinic owners' financial clarity is limited to a report card – tax filing – presented by an accountant that shows figures representing how well that business has done at the end of the year (in relation to what the government wants to know about what you owe in taxes).

Admittedly, in the first few years of my business ownership, I was certainly in that category. I had a detailed report card every twelve months, but I knew nothing about my business and where we went right or wrong. That report cards keeps you legal, but it doesn't do much else. And if it wasn't for a legal requirement from the government, even this process might not happen.

I'm sure you will agree that this numbers thing would be much easier if the report card from your bookkeeper or CPA came with some kind of explanation as to what the heck it all means other than how much money you need to pay the government. Wouldn't it be nice if for just one year your CPA would take the time to sit and explain what all of the numbers actually mean? And, most importantly, tell you how those numbers can be unraveled into changes to make sure that next year's results are better than this year's? But oh no! They insist on talking to you about things that are in *their* language – tax accounting – and stating facts as though they're obvious.

I used to sit there every year and look at my report and wonder when or if I'd ever figure out what it all meant. I was like a nodding dog agreeing to things I didn't understand.

Accountants speak their own language – it's called "confusion".

It's universally tolerated.

And I really believe they do so just to make sure they feel needed. If they speak "confusion" it means we have to ring them six times to clarify what they meant. It also means they can produce hefty bills that we never expected and definitely didn't want.

Yet there's one thing they seem to be very clear on and that is time – especially when it comes to how long they speak to you on the phone or spend composing an email.

Have you noticed that when it comes to their billable time, they're very precise, yet when it comes to a question about what tax liabilities you might incur, they seen to be very vague and need to give you sixty different possible outcomes, each one costing you more than you budget for and leaving you more confused than before you asked?

I'm yet to receive an invoice from any accountant on either side of the Atlantic who doesn't understand the value of their time. Rounding up the minutes needed to speak to you or writing an email response never seems to be hard for them to do.

Twenty minutes and thirty-two seconds for a phone call about your attempt to save money on a purchase of equipment or a new hire's need for health insurance?

Tell me, who on earth is that good at remembering time? (If only they were that precise at projecting my tax return or savings.) Much like politicians, it's safe to say I am not the biggest fan of accountants. Or lawyers. Don't get me started on those people either.

What's really funny about dealing with your accountant is this: you sit there every year hoping that the next year you might understand their reports. Of course, that never happens. And sadly, this lack of financial clarity is primarily why business profit margins never change.

Like I said, I was guilty of this type of behavior toward my company financials at first. I wouldn't say I lacked financial clarity. It's more accurate to say I was financially ignorant. And I got away with it simply because I was so good at marketing and sales and I was able to manage people at a better level than most.

But I was also lucky.

As one of my business coaches would say, I was a "lucky fool"

I might have been doing well, but I was doing well in spite of myself.

I probably cost myself more than I ever made due to my financial ignorance. The price that I paid for financial ignorance was working harder than I should have for the amount of money I was making. Even if I am making good money, I always consider the price I have to pay. It's always relative to what you give up or put in.

Here, let's put that into perspective: had I been a little more financially savvy, I could have been home at 5 P.M. for dinner every night having made the same amount of money as I did working until way past 8 P.M.

Working until 8 P.M. is great for the ego and to tell your followers on social media – but it's not good for your health or your relationships. To me, it's a clear sign that a business owner isn't doing something right.

The real problem that many owners have is that they see finance as a necessary evil. It's this thing they're forced to handle by the government, so they do it just to stay out of jail. There's no love of doing it, and because the language is complicated – and you're only talking once per year with your accountant – you never feel like you understand it. What's more, it is also nearly always the last function of the business that you realize you need.

First comes marketing, then sales, then staff, and then your focus is on culture, and finally, when you start running out of money, it's the realization that you need some more financial clarity.

But by this point you're so caught up in the day-to-day running or busy work of the clinic – or still treating patients – that you don't have time to do it properly.

You know you need to do it – but you don't carve out the time to do it right and you start on the merry-go-round of changing bookkeepers, hoping that the next one will be better.

If you're lucky, you finally one day realize the bookkeeper wasn't the issue – it was that you didn't know what to ask for and so you got what every other business owner gets: a set of report cards that only bookkeepers and accountants can read.

Basically, more and more confusion.

GET YOUR FREE RESOURCE KIT: PAULGOUGH.COM/LEADERSHIP-RESOURCE

The only solution is mastering finance so you can direct the finance professionals to provide precisely what you need in the format in which you need it. If the input from you isn't clear, their output won't be either.

The other challenge you face is that you're diametrically opposed to doing the things you don't excel at naturally.

In my case, marketing and sales come easily. Operations and finance don't. Those functions require completely different skill sets (hence why you have to hire past your own imperfections).

To overcome this natural predisposition, I decided that I had to go all in on learning finance and obsess over it in the same way I had when I first discovered marketing all those years ago. To my surprise and delight, the more I studied finance, the more I actually enjoyed it. As I learned, and the numbers started to become clear, I wanted to know more and more. And the more I knew about it, the more I felt I was asking better questions that would deliver better answers. With better answers, I make better, more informed decisions. Isn't that what we all want?

I'm still on the journey to learn more about finance and as my group of companies gets bigger, I am finding I need a new depth of understanding of the financials.

At first, I simply needed to understand a profit and loss statement. Now I need a new depth of understanding the key ratios and contribution margins, return on assets, and, most importantly, how I can use the numbers I am looking at to make changes to my team's actions and ultimately change the numbers so they are more appealing.

If things are going well, I want to be able to reinforce good behaviors. If things are not going well, I want to be able to correct bad behaviors that are causing poor results – and improve them fast.

The CEO has a number of important jobs and one of them is to make informed decisions (using financial clarity) that get turned into measurable actions. If you measure it, you can change and improve it. That's an important aspect of your job, summed up in one sentence. The game is to get into that position and to do it as fast as possible.

With that in mind, in this chapter, I'm going to introduce you to seven financial reports and pieces of information that you must have and know how to read. I am sure I'll write an entire book on this one day, but for now this is going to give you a head start on understanding what you should know in order to do your job as the CEO well.

1. Annual Budget

The budget is often done around December, looking at the twelve-month period ahead. This is a set of major assumptions about what you would like to happen in the coming financial year.

You don't really know precisely how the year is going to go, but taking a day or so to consider what you want to happen allows you to create a road map of how you're going to achieve your goals.

The point of the exercise is to think through all of the different things that would have to happen for you to meet your financial goals in the next twelve months. It is slightly different from your bigger growth plan in that your annual budget looks only at the next twelve months, whereas your growth plan could cover the next three to five years.

The annual budget is guided by your strategic intent and your primary objective.

When you do the budget, sit down and consider your annual financial target, along with how much income would be needed in specific months and how much you're willing to allocate to expenses. This gives you a more condensed, intense road map to follow.

Admittedly, at first it is difficult to do, as it always feels like you are "guessing." And in the beginning, you are doing just that to a certain degree. But the more you do it, the more accurate it gets.

If you are wrestling with the guessing game when creating a budget, remember that it's not about what *will* happen – it's what you *want* to happen.

Here's the phrase to remember: if you can't make it work on paper first, you will *never* make it work in reality. Use your budget to make sure that your income minus the expenses you're projecting adds up to a number that supports the financial target you want for your business. It doesn't get more complicated than that – it's often only complicated by overthinking it.

2. Cash Flow Forecast

In a fast-growing business – one that is starting to employ more and more people – nothing is more important than doing a rolling thirteen-week cash flow forecast.

A cash flow forecast allows you to get a handle on the flow of money in and out of your bank. It is a look thirteen weeks into the future at what your cash position will likely be so you can avoid running out of cash.

Why thirteen weeks? Because it is widely accepted that it takes thirteen weeks to secure funding or a line of credit from the bank if you need cash.

A thirteen-week cash flow forecast allows you to look into the future and consider all of the cash you should be getting in during that time frame

– and get equally clear on how much is going out. At the end of each week, you have a net cash flow that is either positive or negative. Some weeks you will be positive. Some, for example payroll weeks, you might be negative. Doing the cash flow forecast ensures that you know weeks ahead of time if you're going to have enough cash to meet payroll.

A business owner always sweating over meeting payroll is usually one absent of a cash flow forecast. Doing this exercise every week creates a higher level of intensity and focus than any other financial reporting you can do. It gives you great view of your business in real time and you can prioritize the decisions you need to make, such as to increase your marketing efforts, reduce your expenses, move or delay payments, chase down people who owe you money, or start selling more to make more.

As the CEO, this is another tool that allows you to prioritize actions.

If you're going to run out of cash next week, you're not going to be worried about creating a new system or writing up a new process. You're going to get intensely focused on what you can be doing to get cash in the bank. That could be calling past patients, reactivating people who dropped off, or coming up with a new promotion that will create a surge of package buyers who will put cash in your bank.

As the saying goes, you can survive a year without profit, but you can't survive a month without cash. Cash and profit should not be confused. Profit is theory. Cash is fact. A cash flow forecast ensures that cash remains your priority. Cash is king for a reason.

3. Dashboards Reporting Operational Effectiveness (Your "Cockpit")

Where performance gets measured, performance gets improved. Where performance is reported, performance improves dramatically. Where performance is improved and people can see it, performance improves exponentially.

Said differently, if you want to improve your team, you need dashboards that display how well they're doing and you need to share those dashboards with them.

Dashboards are vital. Dashboards organize data and turn it into information that gives you clues about where you can improve. Having a dashboard displaying the critical drivers of your business is a way of being able to manage your staff for higher performance.

If you want to move from high maintenance to high performance, get a dashboard that shows you objectively what is happening in your business so you can tackle it head on and without emotion.

Politics and drama exist in companies where performance isn't measured objectively. You show me a practice that is riddled with politics and tension and I'll show you a business owner who doesn't have these types of dashboards set up. This is how you stop the office politics and take the emotion out of any conversations you're having with your team about things you need them to do better.

As I mentioned earlier, in my clinic, and in all of my businesses, and now in the practices I consult with via my coaching company, I affectionately call my dashboard the "cockpit." It is a tool that I have created to show me all of the major performance levers in the companies.

I call it the cockpit as a reference to a pilot needing to see all of the dials to be able to fly the plane safely.

My cockpit alerts me to when I am having issues in my clinic with arrival rates being low, or patient cancels being high, or leads being down, or even if our digital marketing has dropped below the agreed standard.

When I see any of the cells turn red – meaning the performance has dropped below what I need to achieve my financial target – then I am able to do something about it. It could be a conversation with the person responsible, offering a suggestion on how to remedy the situation, or, as is usually the case, simply pointing out to the person responsible some basic ways of handling the phone calls that they might have missed or forgotten. Making a fix isn't that difficult. The difficulty is knowing *what* to fix. And with my own "cockpit," I can literally fly my plane – that is, run my clinic – from 3,500 miles away and still have a handle on what is going on and offer advice when needed.

4. Profit and Loss Statement

A profit and loss statement – sometimes called an "income statement" or "P&L" – is a report that tells you how well your business performed in the previous month or year.

It shows the income that you've produced minus the expenses you incurred. What you're left with is the net profit. This is the typical report that is prepared by a bookkeeper and possibly the one you're most familiar with. You usually get it two or three weeks after the previous month ended and then again after the year is over. It is usually what is filed by your accountant with the government in order to work out your taxes.

The profit and loss report is the most basic of reports. Although helpful, it is what is called a "lagging indicator" (your dashboard is a leading indicator) because it tells you what has already happened. It only provides you with a rear-view look at what has happened in the company (whereas your dashboard tells you what is likely to happen in the future). The downside is that it really only confirms what has already happened. It doesn't give you the answers – it should be the start of the questions that allow you to translate the numbers and determine what did or didn't happen in the last month (or year).

5. Budget Versus Actual Report (Variance Analysis)

This is one of my favorite reports. It shows, side by side, what you *wanted* to happen (your budget) and what *did* happen (the profit and loss).

Essentially, it shows you the gap between where you wanted to be and where you ended up. When you get this report, it might show you that you budgeted for making $100,000 in revenue in a month, but you only made $80,000.

That means you have a negative variance of $20,000.

For one month, you might be able to tolerate this.

But if you have too many more months of missing the target, then you've got no chance of making your annual target. You also get to see how much you had budgeted on expenses versus what you spent. If you planned $25,000 for payroll but ended up spending $30,000, it's not going to be long before you blow the budget. Importantly, it also allows you to ask why you spent an extra $5,000, and because you can see the two side by side – your planned versus your actual – you get to see month to month how the company is performing against your expectations.

GET YOUR FREE RESOURCE KIT: PAULGOUGH.COM/LEADERSHIP-RESOURCE

I highly recommend you get this report if you haven't already. Everything in business should be measured – even your own assumptions that were made in the original budget.

6. Accounts Receivable Report

Bluntly, this tells you how good you are at getting the money you're owed – something that most business owners are not very good at!

Truth is, they're just not focused on it or intentional about it.

Surprisingly, getting money that is owed is usually an afterthought that is always playing second fiddle to making more of it. But when you can't get money in (i.e., from an insurance company) then what is the point of producing more bills? This is the fastest way to run out of money and often happens in the rapid growth phase of business. The focus is on making more money – forgetting that there's a second requirement to making it, and that's getting it (the third is keeping it).

In most businesses, chasing money usually happens long after it should have been done. It is usually weeks or months after a bill has been sent out that someone might actually chase it down to find out why it hasn't been paid. Of course, when you do eventually call to find out why it hasn't been paid, you get the usual responses like, "We didn't get the invoice" or "You just missed this month's payment run – it'll be on the next one."

Think about this: if you were as good about getting money in as you were at letting it go, how much cash would you have right now? Or perhaps it needs to be the other way around – what if you were as slow at spending it as you are at asking for it? What would your cash position look like?

If you're a traditional insurance clinic, your accounts receivable (or aged debtors report, as it is called in some countries) is something you should obsess over. "Who's got my money and when am I getting it?" is the first question I ask in every one of my companies on a Monday morning.

If you show any contempt or disrespect to money, I believe it will show you just as much contempt or disrespect back. Fall out of love with it – and it'll fall out of love with you. However, give it your top priority – and it seems to want to prioritize you. That's why they say money flows. And it does – to people who actually want it enough to focus on getting it.

Remember this: money is the oxygen you need to run your clinic – don't ignore your accounts receivable process. And here's a huge tip on this subject – make sure the person who is in charge of chasing it is *not* a "nice" person. I'm serious. You want someone in charge of collecting your cash who is a bit of a "bulldog" and doesn't really care what people think about them. All they care about is getting your money in on time.

7. Balance Sheet

A balance sheet is another one of the legal reports that you're required to produce. A balance sheet shows the strength of your company and tells you the level of assets, debts, and owners' equity. It comes in handy when you're looking to borrow money from the bank or seeking an investor. It is usually the first thing they will look for to see how "credit worthy" your company is and if you have enough assets to cover the note you might be requesting. If you don't have this, expect your level of interest rate to go up when borrowing.

In our type of business, the asset is usually cash – unless you've bought the building your clinic is housed in. Your balance sheet is an important financial document that any serious business owner will have on hand. Be sure to make sure you have one if you plan on growing or borrowing any money from the bank.

So there you go, all of the financial reports and why you need them. I could write an entire book on the financial responsibility of top CEOs – perhaps I will? – but for now, that gives you an introduction to it so that you can get started.

The last thing I'll say on the subject is this: most small clinics stay small because they have an *unprofessional* finance department or a complete lack of respect for the impact that finance, run correctly, can have on their ability to make better decisions. Finance is where the best decisions are made – not your gut. Sure, your subjective view of the business is important. But that must be considered with facts. Emotions nearly always lure you into a false sense of security that rarely ends well. When facts and emotion collide, facts always seem to win.

If you've been avoiding getting financial clarity simply because you don't like the numbers you're seeing, think about this: it's always the business owners who *don't* look at their numbers who really *need* to look at their numbers. And the ones who might be excused for not checking their numbers – because they're doing really well – are the ones who are checking them relentlessly.

Interesting how that little paradox works, isn't it?

Ultimately, as a CEO, you've got to want to look forward to seeing the numbers – good or bad. It's part of your job. Don't take the job if you don't want to do what is required. Don't take the position if all you want is the title. And equally, don't spend your whole business career saying

GET YOUR FREE RESOURCE KIT: PAULGOUGH.COM/LEADERSHIP-RESOURCE

that you're not very good with numbers. You absolutely can figure out the numbers and what they mean – you just have to invest time and perhaps money learning how to do so.

From my own experience, I can tell you it is a fun journey to go on, and if you are searching for a feeling of being "more in control" of your practice, this is how you will find it.

*As an aside, if you're interested in learning more about these types of financial reports and getting real financial clarity, I teach all of this – and more – in depth at my Strategic Planning Workshop, which is available in person and can also be instantly downloaded online. Please send an email to paul@paulgough.com for more information. My team will be happy to hear from you and tell you more about both options.

RECRUIT A PLAYERS AND BUILD THE TEAM

Every business owner will privately admit that they would like "better staff." Many currently believe the only thing holding them back from more success is finding the elusive "A players" they hear about or read about in business books. But no matter what they do, they're nowhere to be found "in their town."

What's the secret to finding these A players?

It's simple: find the *time* to look.

Prioritize your day and your week to put finding and recruiting top performers at the top of your list. I know you're likely to be "busy" – but how can anything be more important than finding people to help you execute the growth plan you've created? I don't think there is. In fact, I firmly believe that recruitment is the most underestimated and overlooked role of a CEO.

Many business owners view "people" and the recruitment process in general as a hassle. As a result, they recruit people who give them a hassle.

Through this chapter and the one that follows, I will encourage you to change your view of hiring. Move away from thinking that it is just about hiring people to do a job.

Stop thinking about putting up a job ad and then paying someone to come to work for you. It's much more important than that. It's about creating a team of the right people who, collectively, allow you to build the type of business you can be proud of. And just as important, one that you can actually walk away from any time you have something else you want to do or somewhere to go.

I've heard it said that you should be careful of the values you choose, for your values dictate the problems you will get in your life.

It's similar with hiring people.

Be careful of the people you choose to employ, for these people will ultimately decide the problems you'll face every day. They'll also limit or enhance the life choices you have available to you. It's difficult to take that three-week trip to Europe you've always dreamed of when you don't have the right staff to run the practice in your absence.

It's quite powerful when you think of it this way, isn't it? It helps to never forget that the people you are looking for are ultimately going to dictate the quality of life you've got.

To be successful at hiring, you need to find people who are aligned with your values and who have the skills you need to solve the problems that being in business creates. It's also about finding people capable of raising the average of the people you've already got. If you're going to bring someone in, why not bring in someone who raises the standard on the people you've already got?

Like anything important in your life, it also needs time allocated to it. When you realize it's one of your most important jobs as a CEO, it's easier to feel at ease with allocating time in your calendar to ensure you do it right.

I know that, privately, most clinic owners dread the hiring process. I believe one of the reasons is that hiring involves people and the erratic tendencies and actions – not to mention the often-unpredictable emotions – they bring to your life as their boss. It is, of course, much easier to focus on the logical aspect of fixing hip pain or helping someone move their leg again after surgery.

But you can't grow a business without people.

All of your leverage is in people.

Having the right people around you lets you get more done with less of your own time invested. That is leverage. When you get more of the right things done, you grow. And really, with hiring, that is all you are doing. You are buying time. You're paying someone to do something that you can't currently get done, or to do work that is now beneath your pay grade as a CEO.

Look, don't take that the wrong way. Nothing is really beneath your pay grade as a CEO. You should be willing and prepared to do *anything* in your practice. It's often how many of us start. But you can't seriously tell me that answering the phone or even, dare I say it, continuously treating patients is the best way for a practice owner to spend all of his time?

Any time your clinic has reached a plateau, look at it more closely and you'll realize that it usually coincides with you running out of time in your day to get things done. What's more, that running out of time likely happened about three to six months before your practice stopped growing. The bottleneck for growth is nearly always you, the practice owner, not being able to prioritize your time.

It's why I keep saying throughout this book that one of the skills you must hone is the ability to prioritize and allocate resources. Time, money, and people are your top three resources. How you use each one determines how successful you are.

BUY BACK TIME

One way to stop your clinic from getting stuck is to stop thinking about "needing to hire people" and instead replacing that with the idea that you're buying back time by replacing yourself.

Start thinking about *wanting* to hire someone so that you can remove yourself from doing things that are not the best use of your time. As a CEO, you're always looking at your day and your week and asking if what you're doing is something someone else should be doing. You're consciously aware of your tasks and looking for things that have somehow crept into your day that shouldn't be there. Why? So that you can be sure you are prioritizing your own time – and your team's – correctly.

Here's a great question: What would it be like if I could give you another forty hours in your week? Stop and think about it for a moment.

I bet you would get so much more done, right? I bet if you wrote it all down, you would have a list as long as your arm of things that you would get done if you suddenly had more time. Well, go ahead and do it. Write them down. What you will find on that list is a number of things that you know you need to do to get to the next level.

Understand this: all of those things you wrote down are what you will need to be able to accomplish if you want to keep growing. If you keep treating patients, answering the phone every time it rings, fighting fires, and always having to replace your people, you'll never grow sustainably. Your clinic is going to stay where it is.

Just look at what you *could* be doing and try to quantify it.

Then ask yourself this question: If that work you know you need to do was actually done – and done well – what would the monetary return be? How much would it be worth to you?

When you know what the fiscal amount would be, then you can calculate the return on investment that you will need to make. The investment is usually a person with a salary requirement you will need to pay. But the amount you're paying out is not what you look at. It is what the *return* will be for paying it out.

For example, if the employee costs you $50 per hour but frees you up to do work valued at $150 per hour, why would you hold back from hiring?

THE PHENOMENON OF "A PLAYERS" WHO TURN OUT TO BE "Z LISTERS"

So that's one way to think about recruitment. And hopefully that gives you some encouragement – and an objective, less emotional way to think about hiring.

Next, let's see if we can alleviate another all-too-common fear that often comes true for business owners: the perennial situation of interviewing someone and you being certain you have found an "A player" or a "rock star" who turns out to be a "Z player" or, as I affectionately call them, a complete "dummy."

Once you've experienced this a few times, it can really put you off hiring for life and cause you to delay recruitment longer than you should. Remember this, though: the decision and the need to hire are different from the person you hired. The decision to hire can be right – and the execution of it poor. But that doesn't mean the original decision to hire wasn't correct. It likely was. Don't back out of hiring altogether just because the first person didn't turn out right. Sometimes you have to kiss a few frogs to find your prince.

The first thing to clear up is this: "A players" aren't found in an interview. "A players" reveal themselves over a number of weeks, months, and even years of working in your company. I literally shudder when I hear a practice owner tell me they did an interview and they found their "rock star." How can you know that from an interview?

The reality of a successful interview process is that you have nothing more than the *potential* for an A player. During the interview process, you're assuming, based on the data you collected during the process, that they *could* be an A player. The key word is *assuming*.

And what's more, just because they were an A player for someone else, and came with a glowing reference from someone else, that does not mean they are going to be an A player for you. Why? Simply because you're going to have very different standards and values than their last boss. At least, you better! You have to have your own set of standards and values that, when achieved and matched, means your people are able to call themselves a success on your job.

Over time, whether or not they can achieve those standards consistently and reliably – without any fuss, drama, or headaches – is how you get to decide whether you have an A player or a rock star on your hands (or a perpetual pain in the ass who consistently frustrates more than delights).

A problem for many when it comes to recruitment is that they're blindsided by great interviewees. Myself included. I've made many a "great decision" to hire someone only to realize two weeks later that the person I interviewed was a fraud – or he was a great actor.

The person I interviewed went into the phone booth after we met and changed from Superman back into Clark Kent on his worst day. The person I interviewed disappeared and an imposter arrived.

More than once, I've been blinded by an interviewee's willingness to solve my business's often-urgent need. The biggest mistake is in believing the first person who tells you they "loved the sound of the role" and that it was "just what they were looking for."

How many times have you come out of a bad relationship with an employee and caught yourself saying, "But they said they liked to sell"? (Even though they later refused to even pick up the phone). Or, "They told me they knew how to do Google ads"? (Yet it turns out they don't know a Google ad from a job ad.) Then there's my personal favorite, "They told me they were a detail-orientated person." (Yet they seemed to develop an acute case of amnesia once they started working for you.)

I've done it many times.

The problem is that what people say and what they do are often very different things. What people think about themselves and their reality are often miles apart. Humans are great at criticizing and finding fault with others – but we're not so good at doing it for ourselves.

We're also sometimes a little inconsistent with our words and actions.

People say they want to lose weight – just as they're about to order their fourth pizza in five days. Heck, people stand on the altar and say "I do" to loving and being with someone for the rest of their lives and then a year later change their minds.

Reality check: people desperately want to fit in and desperately want to be liked and they'll do anything and say anything to make that happen – including altering the truth about themselves in an interview.

ASK WHY YOU SHOULDN'T HIRE THIS PERSON

When in doubt, err on the side of caution. And if you find yourself perennially hiring "Z listers" (who pose as A listers), start coming out of interviews and asking yourself these questions:

1. "If I had another five candidates to interview, would I be even considering this person?"
2. "Is this definitely the right person for the role, or could I be settling for having my recruitment headache solved rather than continuing to look for the right person?"
3. "What are five reasons I should *not* employ this person?"
4. "When this person leaves my company, what will be the reasons? Do I already see those signs now?"

Incidentally, I wrote an entire book on interviewing and the whole recruitment process. You can get that book, *The Physical Therapy Hiring Solution: How to Recruit, Hire and Train World-Class People You Can Trust*, at wwww.paulgough.com/books. The book outlines the entire outcomes-based process for finding the people that you need to grow a company that does not rely constantly upon the owner.

For now, though, and until you read that book, know that the real secret to successful hiring is that you must *always be looking* for great talent. A great CEO always has a stack of resumés on his or her desk. There are names of people you know who could step into any role in your practice should anyone on your staff want or need to leave. They could also take the place of anyone you consider a "flight risk" who could leave your business vulnerable or exposed.

SO, WHO ARE THESE "A PLAYERS" CANDIDATES?

Let's move on to getting clear on *who* you should be hiring and *where* to find them. What do A players look like? And where are they all hiding? Well, these elusive candidates that you're always looking for are hiding in plain sight. They're right in front of you – you just have to know how to spot them. They're not wearing camouflage or a Harry Potter-style invisibility cloak. They're regular people who are doing exceptionally good things by leveraging a simple set of qualities and character traits that make them valuable to employers like you and me.

The key to finding more great candidates is to know, understand, and recognize the qualities that make them great employees. Here are what I've noticed to be the most important:

1. Accountability

The first and most important quality is **accountability**. The best employees love to be held accountable. The winners in life are people who want to be told how they're doing and what they need to do to improve further. Sadly, accountability is something that most people run from as they get older. They get to a certain age and believe that accountability is not needed now that they're an adult.

We're living in an entitlement culture with the socialist idea that everyone should be given everything for free (without having to work for it). Accountability is becoming a lost concept that most people would struggle to spell, let alone understand.

And it's sad that it's happening that way.

Think about how most people's lives go. The most successful period of their lives — and nearly always the happiest — is when they were kids.

What do kids have an abundance of?

That's right, accountability!

They're accountable to their parents and their schoolteachers. They are constantly told by their teachers via tests where they rank in terms of performance. A report card at the end of the year tells them what they need to do next year to improve. Their parents are constantly holding them accountable for managing time, being polite, and other standards of living that are in line with how they want their children to be raised.

People achieve more as kids than they do at any other time of their lives because there is so much accountability baked into their lives. As I said right at the outset of this book, a parent is simply a coach who holds their children accountable for better standards than the children could achieve on their own.

Ironically, kids often hate every bit of it and it's usually the first thing any young adult wants to break free from in favor of a carefree way of living that is mistaken for independence. The initial freedom felt from not being held accountable to anyone or anything is ecstasy — and some people never have another day of accountability in their lives. It's sad that they don't recognize the void that has been left.

This leads so many people to see accountability as criticism or a way of attacking who they are in some way. And because you need accountability to grow your company, I think this general dislike of accountability is one of the biggest challenges you are up against as an employer.

But believe me, there are people out there who will relish your accountability. There are people who are desperate to know how they're doing and what they can do to improve. In fact, there are people who will leave you if you don't give it to them.

In your interview process, you should be asking them questions about accountability and how their previous bosses handled it. If they say they've never been held accountable to anyone before or they give you the "I hold myself to my own high standards" line, then you're on rocky ground. You are not looking at a future hall of famer for your practice. You're likely looking at a liability. This is someone who will start well, but the minute you ask them why their performance isn't where it should be, they'll accuse you of being too demanding and quit.

Now, hopefully, they leave sooner rather than later as the cost of keeping them is going to be way more than whatever you've invested in them so far. But even if they leave fairly quickly, you've still got to go back to find someone to replace them. This is where you lose momentum. This is when your practice growth starts to slow down. When you're constantly replacing people who slipped through the interview process net, it is costly in more ways than one. It sure pays to get it right first time.

2. Commitment

An A player will bring a level of **commitment** that exceeds most others. If they're not committed, it does not matter how good they are at answering the phone or treating a bad back. They'll be toxic for your business and cause you to always feel like you're treading on egg shells – waiting for the next kick off.

By that, I mean they'll do a good job for a period of time – usually when things are good, or conditions are stable – but they'll always be the one who kicks up a fuss the minute the playing field changes or the tide turns against you.

As soon as you need them to step up and do some overtime or work on a Saturday, they remind you it isn't in their contract or what you agreed to in writing. They'll tell you they have to see their kid play sports on the weekend – even though they've done it for the last fifty-one weeks in a row. They're not willing, or committed, enough to give it up just this once to help the company out.

And by the way, I respect the people who do that. I just can't have them in my world. I need a little flexibility in every role and an employee's commitment should never be in question. I am 100 percent committed to paying my staff's wages each month. I am not flexible about that. They don't have to beg me to pay them each month, so why should I have to beg them for commitment to achieving the outcome we agreed upon in the interview?

Look for people who both *say* they are committed and *show* they are committed.

3. Coachable

A players are **coachable**. We spoke about this at length earlier in the book, but it is worth revisiting under the banner of a CEO's role. If they're not accountable, they're a waste of time. If they're not committed, you're going to have a headache that comes and goes as frequently as the weather changes in Britain.

But if they're not coachable, you're just plain stuck.

That's because the only way anyone or any company can grow is if the people in your company are willing to improve and grow. You don't do that merely by spending more time on Earth or with "experience."

That really is fantasy-land stuff – and something I wish I had realized much earlier in life. Just because someone is older than me, that doesn't mean they are wiser. It *could* mean they are, but not *just* because they were born a few years or decades before me. It is a ridiculous, yet commonly accepted, belief that people are cleverer just because they're older.

You only improve your performance in anything if you get intentional about improving it. That starts with coaching. It doesn't have to be the type of coaching that you would assume a runner or swimmer is getting to win the Olympics – but the principle isn't far off.

The coach, knowing precisely what Michael Phelps or Usain Bolt wants to achieve, and by when, observes what their student is doing and then makes daily recommendations on how to improve what they're doing in order to get there. That's it. That's coaching. No real magic.

If the student is committed and they're willing to be held accountable, magic often happens in the form of results and accolades. It is no different anywhere else in your life.

Even as a business owner, I am the product of my accountability, my commitment, and the coaching I invest in. I am a product of all that. If I deem it important to me and helping me get to where I want to be, then it has to be the same for the people around me. It can't be true for me and yet somehow my employees are exempt. The only reason that their jobs exist is because I embrace all of these things. It must be so that they do the same to some degree otherwise my company will lack a dedication to the values that you believe in.

As you read this, you must consider these principles to be true for you.

If you want to be an equivalent A player or rock star CEO, you will not get there without all three of these things in place. Ask yourself:

Who is coaching you?

Are you getting any *real* business coaching?

Are you being held accountable?

Or do you think you're beyond that now that you've been in business for ten years? I've seen many once-successful business owners fall short of achieving their full potential because they neglected accountability in their lives or removed themselves from coaching programs because they'd heard it all before or wanted "something new."

The problem is they'd never perfected or mastered the "something old".

New is tempting. New has sex appeal attached to it. It can also be distracting and is more often than not just a better-marketed version of something you already knew – but just neglected to do or forgot.

Great coaching never lets you lose sight of the basics and how important they are to you ever getting to the point where the complex becomes relevant.

It makes sense to master walking before you can run. The problem is that there's a big difference between common sense and common practice. Great coaching helps you to put common things into daily practice and get lasting results.

If you want the A player at your company, do what is needed of A player CEOs. You need to walk the walk, not just talk the talk.

4. Shared Values

Aside from being accountable, coachable, and committed, something else you need to find in your people is **shared or common values**. All of the best relationships last because the people involved have values in common. They want and respect similar things. They hold the same things at heart.

In contrast, the worst relationships usually turn out that way because the people involved never stopped to consider that they might like each other, but they don't have values in common. I said it earlier and here's a reminder: choose your values wisely, as values dictate the problems in your life and ultimately therefore the quality of it. They also dictate the quality of every relationship you're in.

At the heart of the best romantic relationships is a sharing of values – not of interests. I do not need to be interested in the same things as Natalie (my partner of fourteen years) for our relationship to work. But I must be on the same page as her when it comes to the things we value.

Examples of shared values in relationships include love, financial security, knowledge, and personal growth. If you're living with someone who likes to gamble or spend the family pay check on booze or drugs, then you've got opposing values. The other person values having a wild time and you want to be more fulfilled and to feel safe. It isn't going to last.

Equally, and this is a challenge I see in small business owners, if you value growth and learning and the person you're living with doesn't, they'll struggle to understand why you're always wanting to invest in yourself or your business. If they value financial security – which many do – you've got opposing values and it will cause a clash from time to time (until they see the additional cash come into the house, of course).

It is the same in business. You are in a 24/7 relationship with your team. Whether that relationship is toxic or hedonistic, it all comes down to values.

Do you and your employees both *really* value learning?

Do they value being prepared for work and willing to be at work fifteen minutes early to prepare, or do they think that work starts at 9 A.M. on the dot? Do they think they're being paid to "warm up" for work?

What about the people you take care of – your customers?

Do your employees treat your business's customers with the same level of respect and courtesy that you do? Have they even got it in them to want to do that, or do they treat the customers great only when they feel great? Do they have to have all of the stars lined up in their personal life for them to bring a happy smile to work? Or will they find a way to leave the issue with their husband at home for nine hours and light up the life of every one of your customers, regardless? Those who *really* value their customers do the latter.

You show me a clinic with a crappy culture full of B and C players and I'll show you a business owner who isn't clear on his or her own personal values. I've said it many times that a business is a reflection of the owner's standards. It is also a reflection of his or her values.

Are you clear on yours?

If you are, during the interview process you can ask questions of your potential employees to see if their values match up to yours. "Tell me about the last thing you learned. What was it and how did it help you?" is a simple question you could ask an interview candidate. If they tell you that the last thing they learned was at school, it is clear you have someone who does not value learning or growth and therefore you're going to have a clash and you will not get them to change. You'll try, but it'll never work.

Human behaviour is consistent 88 percent of the time. Willing someone to learn, or expecting that they should learn, won't work in someone who is absent of the desire to learn.

Back to relationships. All the will in the world doesn't rescue an unhappy marriage. Marriages rarely break down because of a lack of trying. No, they break down in spite of trying and because values were not aligned. It is very rare that anyone changes what they truly value. This is why you cannot change employees. They can only change themselves and it only happens when they alter their values and raise their standards. They may evolve over time, but rarely will they do it because it's what you want. Save yourself the heartache and get this right at the recruitment stage. You'll see how important this is in the chapter on culture.

5. Standards

Standards are next on the list of things you're looking for in A players. It's easy to say that you have high standards, and you may very well have high standards, but the question is: compared to what?

Everyone will tell you in an interview that they have high standards, but what are we comparing them to? High standards in relation to the guy you just fired for not being able to get his backside to work on time consistently? Or high standards that were set working for a previous boss who didn't have standards clearly set?

Again, this is a topic where it's easy to get duped. Businesses that provide great customer service don't need to market that they provide great customer service. They just do it and the client notices. The same is true with potential employees. They don't just tell you they have high standards. They show up with high standards and, ideally, they exceed the standards that you've set.

To look for clues to their standards, I'll often ask questions such as, "When it comes to time keeping, or arriving at work, if your time sheet says 9 A.M. start, what time do you think you should arrive in the office?" What they'll often do is tell you that they like to be early. They'll say that they like to arrive at 8:45 A.M. to be ready for work, or something like "*I'm the type* of person who likes to be at work to get ready to start work. I'm not the type of person to just arrive right at 9 A.M. No, that's not me."

When they say that, you're going to reply "Great, I've written that down as your standard." If I offer you the job, I will remind you of your own standards. If you're ever slipping, I'll politely remind you that you're letting *yourself* down.

This is a completely different way to ensure you're hiring people with high standards. I've learned it isn't just about *my* own standards or what I expect, it's about what the person considers to be *their* standards. Once I know that, my job becomes to hold them to that.

Will their standards drop from time to time? As sure as night follows day. Their standards *will* drop. It's the job of the CEO to spot this – and ensure it does not become a habit (you'll also spot this via the dashboard you should have – the one we discussed in the earlier chapter – that monitors your team's performance.)

Another standard you might choose not to tolerate is the overuse of social media on your time. I have zero tolerance for it. Not because of the time they're spending on it, and not because I think I am paying them while they spend time on it, but because of how long it takes them to get back to being in work mode after being on it.

I will lose money as they come off the platforms and attempt to respond to client emails or answer a phone call from a patient who wants to book an appointment. If they're not switched on, we lose the client. That's where it really costs me money. Another standard is to never miss a deadline – or to do everything possible to ensure customers get what they need in their desired time frame, without excuse.

Raising your standards is the key to all success, both in life and in business. If you can find and recruit people who have standards that are higher than the ones you already have, then you're going to have a very successful business.

In the recruitment process, make sure that you ask questions that reveal the person's standards. Write them down. Bring those standards back out during onboarding, one-on-one conversations, or just from time to time when you think they're dropping the ball. The key to being a liberator and not coming across as a dominator – like we discussed earlier in the book – is to ensure that you're holding them accountable for the standards they hold *for themselves*. These are the standards they've told you about. The standards that got them the job in the first place. Remember, you employed them for a reason – and it wasn't because they appeared to have low standards.

Do this and it's almost impossible for them to argue with you about what it is you're asking of them. Sure, they can say that they don't like you having pointed it out, but they can't say it's not deserved. After all, they told you their standards. You're also taking the position that they're letting *themselves* down – not you or the company. I find that this is a significantly greater motivator to affect change than beating them with a stick about how it's not good enough and I expect more. Liberate, don't dominate.

6. The Right Skills

The candidates that you're looking for do *not* have to have previous experience in your exact role. They must, however, have previous experience using the *skills* you need them to have to be successful in your role. That is a huge difference. It is a big and very clear distinction you must make if you want to open up the candidate pool and give yourself a better chance of finding A players.

Almost every job ad says, "previous experience required." This implies that you must have worked on a front desk for someone else at a medical office – and, if not, you can't do the job. What a load of rubbish. You don't want their experience in that role – you want the skills that they've used. Those skills can be used in multiple roles. The key for the CEO – and what often forms the difference between good and bad CEOs – is understanding what these skills actually are and how they can be used to solve problems in your role.

The front desk person's job might look like it is to sit at the front desk, answer the phone, and greet patients. It might also seem like you'll get a better employee if you can find someone who has done that for twenty years already. But take a closer look and you'll find that the actual role involves things like selling your clinic's value, retaining unhappy clients, being timely and organized, being detail oriented, and having the ability to provide white-hot customer experiences.

When you look at that list, you realize that people in many different fields and industries are doing these things and could be a great fit for what you need.

I often advertise my jobs with the phrase "experience in this exact role is not needed." I get much better candidates. I get people who would never have applied if I didn't say that because, like most, they assume that they won't be suitable for the job because they haven't been an operations manager of a private practice before.

Believe me, it's nearly always true that you don't want someone with previous experience in a medical facility. The standards of service are often dreadful – and they'll be used to keeping phone calls as short as possible. That won't do anything to strengthen the relationship you have with the patients you want to keep for life.

Even a brand new and recently qualified physical therapist has skills that make him suitable. He might not have been a physical therapist at this point, but he should have had a previous job.

What can you learn about him from that job?

If he worked in a bar – surely he had to work for tips? Ask what his average nightly tip rate was compared to his co-workers. This will tell you how good his service is.

Ask him how many nights he worked that job through college – it'll tell you how committed he is. Ask how often he asked for feedback from his superior – it'll tell you how coachable he is. Ask what values he liked about his past boss – he's telling you what his own values are. Ask him how many upsells he made to his customers each night – he's telling you if he's any good at selling or is even comfortable doing it.

The clues are always *in their history*. The interview process is about collecting as many of these clues as possible so you can make the most informed and confident decision.

And what if they've never had a job before? Ask yourself seriously if you want to be their first boss. I wouldn't. If they're 25 years old and have never had a job, I am not sure they're going to be a good fit for how I work. It would take a miracle for us to get along and I'm not sure I believe in miracles. I prefer objective measures of performance and being able to collect data that gives me a reasonable chance of getting the right candidate.

There you go. Those are my thoughts on who you should be looking for – the specific qualities and attributes that the A Players have. But, as you know, finding them is one thing. The million-dollar question is how to keep them. Also, what skills do you need as a leader to really get the best from them? Turn the page to the next chapter and I'll tell you!

HOW TO RETAIN AND COACH A PLAYERS

Building a great team isn't just about putting players on the team – it's about retaining them and helping them evolve so they add value to the team and your company. In essence, you're growing and getting better together.

In the last chapter, I said every employee should raise the average. That won't happen just by them agreeing to a pay structure and showing up on time each day. What's more, just because you pay them what you agree on, that doesn't mean they'll stay. That's why I want to bring your focus to the importance of retaining your A players – and how to do it.

How do you keep your A players happy? It's simple – as simple as asking them what it will take to keep them. As in, what conditions and circumstances need to be in place for them to consider staying? Retaining them starts in the interview process when you ask them something like this: "If I give you the job, it is because I see someone with the *potential* to be an A player for my company. Assuming that is true, I would want to keep you for many years. What would I have to do to keep you at my company?"

Then, just be quiet and let them speak.

They'll tell you what you have to do. They'll tell you how they need to be treated in order for them to hang around with you. I keep saying this, and I'll say it throughout this book. You have a relationship with your staff. It can be a good one or a not-so-good one. But you still have one.

Like any relationship, you need to work on it. And for it to have any chance of lasting, *you've* got to know what they want *you* to do.

Think about your romantic relationship.

Imagine if, at the start, you both wrote down what you're specifically looking for in the relationship in order to stay together.

Maybe you did, and that is why you're still together. But sadly, most people don't do that. And if they did, they are mostly talking about things like how many kids they'll have or a certain type of house or a desired standard of living. Fine. But those are not the things that cause the relationship to break down (or last).

Many couples get the kids, the house, and the exotic vacations, but the relationship doesn't always last. It's because there are certain other things that need to be adhered to in order for it to last. Usually it comes down to shared values and whether or not someone feels like they're making progress in their life (which is a by-product of the relationship that you're in).

It's my experience that when you ask an employee this question – "What has to happen to keep you?" – they don't talk about money. Most don't even say that they need good career opportunities. No. They list things that are way more important than that. The things employees want are always at the values level of life.

WHAT YOUR EMPLOYEES REALLY WANT FROM YOU

One of the things employees want is to be **respected**. They want to feel admired for what they're doing for you. If it isn't there, they'll begin to wonder why not. Everyone has a set of qualities and abilities. It isn't always the case that the qualities or the abilities they have are actually what you need for your business, but that doesn't mean they can't be or shouldn't feel respected as human beings.

Every employee has personal qualities that you have to look for and find. Even if the relationship doesn't work out, be respectful about how it ends. Don't embarrass people or try to make an example of them on the way out (unless they steal from you, of course, in which case it is a public hanging). How they leave your world sets the tone for how much other members of the team respect you – or are able to feel respected by you.

I try to end all of my relationships with exiting staff on as good of terms as possible. Some members of my team have quite literally frustrated the life out of me – but in the end I've sat and offered my phone number and the ability to call me any time they ever need someone to talk to about anything they're going through.

If someone quits, I never take any of it personally. In fact, it's very rare that I react to it. I always try to put some distance between finding out that someone is leaving and when I actually speak to them about it.

That gives me a much better opportunity for a conversation where I can find out more about why they're leaving – and even reverse the decision if they are having second thoughts (and assuming I want them to stay.) Either way, whether I asked someone to leave or they chose to, there's no need for the level of respect between two people to drop just because the employee-boss relationship didn't work out or they wanted to go in a different direction.

The other thing employees will tell you is that they want to feel **valued**. They need to feel important and they need to feel as though they're doing something beneficial for the company.

People who are lacking a feeling of being valued are, in effect, lost. What is more, as soon as they feel lost, you're losing them from your company. When they lose their feeling of being valued, they're likely already looking for other jobs. They'll tell you that your job isn't "doing it for them" anymore, but really it was never the job – it was always that they didn't feel valued. When they lose that, they're missing a feeling of fulfilment. It's difficult to live without fulfilment because it causes people to constantly question if they're in the right place and doing the right thing.

And even if they stay, if they're constantly questioning if they're in the right place, you're never getting their best performance. That leads to conversations about sloppy or poor work and that sets in play a series of challenging conversations that lead to the employee being disheartened. Because they're always being berated (for poor performance), they now don't feel valued. They don't feel respected and they begin to connect the role and your company with their feeling crappy. None of this was needed. All that was needed was some kind of conversation to close the gap between the person feeling valued and the owner showing it.

Simple stuff when you can recognize it (which, admittedly, is not always easy to do).

The other thing that A players crave? **Coaching**. Seriously, the A players crave improvement. If you don't value it or are not willing to do it, someone like me will. I love to and often do collect A players who stay with me for years because I am the first one to provide the type of coaching – life and business – that has been missing in their lives since they stopped getting it from school or parents.

Coaching is non-negotiable in the life of an A player (it should also be non-negotiable in the life of a CEO!).

If you ever tell me you've got A players, the first thing I'll do is ask you about the level of desire and anticipation these people have for information and personal growth. If you can't tell me, I know you don't have a real A player. Truth is, you might have a very good B+ player, but not a true A player. You have Scottie Pippen, but you don't have Michael Jordan. And that's fine. Even the great Chicago Bulls of the '90s needed some great B+ players, but they didn't win the championship the years the A+ player was missing.

If you want your A players to hang around, you need **to respect** them, make them feel **valued,** and provide a level of **coaching** that they're not going to get anywhere else. Providing all three makes it very difficult to walk away if they're ever tempted to leave you for money elsewhere. They're risking not getting everything you provide at the next place. They might get more money or a few extra perks, but these three are what your best performers really need and likely can't get from the big, crappy mill-like health care practices you're competing with for their loyalty.

Respect, a feeling of being valued, and coaching are no match for sleep pods, breakfast on tap, being allowed to bring your dog to work, or even Taco Tuesday in the office (or whatever else companies try to do to manufacture culture these days).

Now don't get me wrong, you *do* still have to pay them well – but what I am absolutely adamant about is that *just* paying them well doesn't make them stay. The two are not mutually exclusive and that means someone else could provide them both. It needs to be you. Once you have them, don't lose them over not providing these most fundamental and basic things.

GET YOUR FREE RESOURCE KIT: PAULGOUGH.COM/LEADERSHIP-RESOURCE

OTHER FACTORS INVOLVED IN RETAINING A PLAYERS

Those three things we just discussed are just the tip of the iceberg when it comes to keeping your best performers. Asking them what they want – and delivering on it consistently – is just the first step in keeping them. Other things also need to happen as well.

1. Can They Call Themselves Successful?

Ultimately, the litmus test for staff staying in their role is whether or not they are able to call themselves successful. If they are coming to work every day and they're not feeling success, pretty soon they're going to connect their low moods to the job.

When any new employee starts with me, I tell them that I will do everything I can to ensure they can call themselves successful in their job. It's my obligation to at least make sure that I do everything I can to make that happen. If they do the same, and assuming I haven't been lied to in the interview process, we have a chance of them being able to label themselves a success (in the role).

Remember, though, that any job must come with a clearly defined set of standards and a scorecard that shows them what success looks like. They're a success according to your *pre-agreed* definition. This definition is established during the recruitment process when you spelled out what success looked like and they acknowledged that they fully understood.

Success for a physical therapist could be that all patients convert to a plan of care, that patients stay on schedule and never leave, that every patient refers another, or that they rate your practice nine out of ten or higher on customer service satisfaction surveys. The definition cannot be vague. The clearer the better. The clearer it is, the easier it is for them to achieve, and therefore be able to call themselves a success.

Being successful absolutely cannot be claimed just because they worked hard.

Nor can it be achieved just because they showed up or, worse still, they didn't show up with an "attitude" like the last one did (the one they replaced). Those might be the standards that big institutions have accepted or settled for – but we need more than that. Unlike the government, we don't have a federal reserve that lets us print more money when we screw up recruitment.

2. Does The Company's Growth Justify Keeping Them?

It sounds elementary, but one of the reasons growth is justified is to be able to keep the people you've got. The best people are always going to want to be around the energy that comes with growth and they'll want to see that opportunities are being created. Growth is exciting and the best people want to be part of that excitement.

Plus, your best people will continuously expect to be compensated more than they are right now – whatever pay grade they're at. If your company isn't growing its profitability, then each time you get asked for a pay raise, you have to either give it to them and instantly become less profitable or reject it and risk losing them.

There are plenty of reasons to want to grow. One of them is just to avoid getting left behind. Even with a growth rate of 10 percent year over year, chances are you're not growing fast enough to keep up with your team's collective wage demands. A 20 percent increase in profitability

GET YOUR FREE RESOURCE KIT: PAULGOUGH.COM/LEADERSHIP-RESOURCE

year over year is the number to shoot for to allow you to keep everyone happy. Yourself included.

3. Do the B Players Irritate the A Players?

If cash is king, then culture is queen. You don't often realize that until a bad one starts developing, but trust me, the culture you grow is going to determine how long your true A players hang around.

I say *true* A players. That is because people who are good at their jobs – yet are a poor culture fit – are not true A players. Being good at your job gets you the job. Being a good culture fit helps you keep your job. This type of "good at the job" – but "pain in the ass" – employee is often tolerated by employers too focused on what they might lose if the employee leaves.

It is only when the employee leaves that they realize they were losing twice over because of the negative impact that person was having on the rest of the team. Ten other team members who reduce their output by as little as 10 percent is going to cost you a lot more than any one person can make up on their own. Fact.

It isn't just about the amount of money they bring in. If they push back or kick up a fuss every time you want to introduce a new policy or procedure, the frustration and amount of time wasted trying to convince them to cooperate stifles your creativity as a CEO. Right then and there, you're losing more money that you can ever realize. A players don't cause you headaches or give you heartache every time they don't agree with a new policy or procedure you'd like to implement. Trust me, after twelve years and more than seventy staff, I can tell you that the team members you will call A players *do not* back you into a corner.

No, they back you to the hilt.

They might ask a couple of questions about it just to be clear in their own head, and that is okay, but they'll ultimately agree to support you. These are the people you want around you – for life. They are there to support you and they learn to love your new ideas and can't wait to implement a price increase because they know it's good for the company.

Never keep people who don't back you.

This is a non-negotiable rule in all of my companies.

My employees can disagree with things – they can raise concerns and questions – but they have to back me once the decision is made. We have to agree to not know enough and trust that what we're doing is for the greater good of the company and the target *I* set. That's my privilege as the business owner and founder and can never be lost on anyone in the company.

Final point on this: be careful of how the A players and B+ players view each other. To get the right culture, the A players need to be reminded that they can still learn something from the B+ players. Remind them that B+ players often do the work that goes unnoticed to make the job of the A players glamourous and easy. You need both on the team, but not too many of either to cause conflict or disillusionment.

4. A Leader Who Supports but Challenges

I know we covered this earlier, but it is important enough look at again. Your team needs a leader who supports but challenges them. We don't want to mollycoddle, and we don't want to hold their hands while they're doing everything. There's enough of that going on in society. Eventually, you've got to let your child walk to school on their own.

GET YOUR FREE RESOURCE KIT: PAULGOUGH.COM/LEADERSHIP-RESOURCE

With that said, we also don't want to abdicate. It's about finding that perfect balance of them knowing that you're there for them but ensuring that they have everything they need to do their jobs properly (so they'll never need to reach you even though they can).

Your job is to give them the tools, ensure they have the appropriate resources, and confirm that they know exactly what the outcome looks like – including what time frame you want it to be completed in. Miss any of those things and you're likely to be abdicating or you'll end up micromanaging.

If they do happen to need you or have questions, it should be a conversation that fills in the blanks or provides direction. But it should not end in your doing the job for them. Remember, the best CEOs are able to move things *without* touching them

5. A Safe Workplace Environment

Employees need to feel safe and secure in their workplace. Like any relationship, it is only going to last or be considered a good one if that person feels safe. They need to know that there's not the constant threat of redundancy in the air or an environment that makes them feel vulnerable. People naturally have a lot of insecurities. A workplace that is volatile will do nothing to settle those insecurities.

True story: when I was growing up – mainly in my teenage years – I lived in a home that wasn't exactly what you would call "calm." My parents weren't what you would call a "good fit for each other" when it came to actually getting along. They were married – but they weren't *happily* married.

The house I grew up in might have been calm for a day or two at a time, but rarely longer than that. Don't get me wrong, I had a great childhood. I was very lucky, and I am to this day very thankful for much of it. But the house I lived in wasn't an environment that I would ever wish to go back to. I couldn't and wouldn't thank you for taking me back to the house I grew up in and it was primarily because I didn't always feel safe.

My parents didn't exactly see eye to eye (on pretty much anything) and so I always felt on edge or worried that the house was about to "go up" again for a reason I could never see coming. It wasn't always like that. But I was often walking on eggshells, worrying about what might or might not happen in the house between my parents that night or that weekend.

I don't know which is worse – things actually happening or worrying they will. The more I think about it, it's the latter. After all, fear isn't real.

We lived in a nice house in a nice area of town. It had a front and back garden with four bedrooms. We had two cars and it was very quiet. It was certainly somewhere most people in town would be happy to live. However, I remember saying to my mother on more than one occasion that I would rather leave this "nice" house and live in the worst part of town – just to feel consistently safe in my own home.

In business terms, I was saying that I would rather take a pay cut to go work in a place where I felt safe than stay in a higher-paying job where I felt insecure and constantly vulnerable. Which leads me to the next point:

6. A Leader With Consistent Emotions

If you're unable to keep your own emotions in check, you will not keep any staff – let alone the best ones. And if they do hang around, you don't deserve them. A responsibility I believe that you take on as the leader of the company is to provide a safe environment – much like that of a parent for their children. It's one that your employees can at least feel protected in.

I believe everyone has a right to that at home and at work.

Employees cannot be living in a perpetual state of fear over you losing your temper or getting visibly aggressive because things aren't going well for you. Even if it is their fault, it is still *your* fault because you put them there in the first place (and subsequently kept them there). You're creating the poison and drinking it yourself. That's dumb. And you shouldn't take it out on them just because you don't like the potion you made.

I think this is one of the most underestimated and simultaneously overlooked skills needed in a good CEO. You have to master it if you want to keep A players.

Don't fall foul of copying people like Steve Jobs – who, if you believe the stories, made his employees feel very insecure and unsafe during his *first* stint at Apple, which didn't end well. It ended so badly that he didn't even get a wave good-bye out of the parking lot from any of the employees when he left on his final day. That's how bad it had gotten.

It also coincided with Apple's worst-ever period of time financially.

However, by all accounts, it was very different when he returned for the second spell, mostly because he treated his people better. It also coincided with him creating the most successful company on earth that has employees desperate to work there and never wanting to leave.

Your best employees will not tolerate a boss who isn't able to be consistent with their emotions 99.9 percent of the time. They'll have too many offers to go and work for someone who can. Same in your relationship – if you're flying of the handle all the time and you're living with someone who really values herself, she's not going to hang around with you for long.

Basically, I guess what I am saying is that even though running a business is volatile, scary, lonely, unpredictable, and often costs you more money (and heartache) than you ever get in return, it is still no excuse for being an emotional train wreck at work. You have to get your act together if you want to keep the best staff.

If you are struggling with your emotions at work, understand this: chances are that your volatility at work brings out the worst in your people. This will cause more volatility in you. It can only change if you do.

ESSENTIAL QUALITIES REQUIRED TO COACH AND LEAD A PLAYERS

Now that you know what they want, what skills will help you keep them? I thought long and hard about this and came up with a list of things I think you will need to be able to effectively lead the best employees. This isn't your typical list of things that you might see in other books and I think you will be pleasantly surprised at how simple it is to do this right.

1. Love of Developing People

If A players want coaching, it makes sense, then, that in order to have a chance of keeping them, *you* will need to have a love of coaching and developing people. You're not going to be a good coach if you don't enjoy coaching people and watching them grow.

And, if I dare say it, I don't think many bosses really do. Sure, they'll say they do – but I suspect that is paying lip service to the view that they want people to have of them.

I think many bosses or business leaders are too caught up in achieving targets or the "busyness" of business to ever notice the development of their people.

I also don't believe that most business leaders ever consider this as part of their remit. The common attitude – which is now very outdated – is that an employee gets paid to do their job and that should be enough to keep them happy.

That might have worked during the Great Depression when unemployment was in the 50 percent range, but today, when people can find new jobs on Indeed or Google during their lunch break, it's not going to cut it.

Here's what I would say to every CEO: coaching people and watching them grow shouldn't ever be just about keeping *them* happy. It should also be about your *own* personal level of happiness that you get from doing it. That brings fulfilment, which is one of the most powerful and rewarding feelings you can ever get.

2. Time

How much time do you have to give them? They don't always need you – but they should always feel like they can reach you. I live 3,500 miles away from my sister in the UK – but I bet she feels like she can always get me any time she needs me. It should be the same with your staff.

Pretending to be too busy to be bothered is a disease that will kill your company. You are Superman in their eyes, and you should always have time available.

Now here's the distinction I need to make: I do *not* believe in having an open-door policy. No way. That kills the productivity and creativity of a CEO as you end up fighting fires. If you're not careful, you breed dependence when what you're really trying to create is independence.

There should be a formal process where they can reach you and are able to schedule time with you that suits you both. Nothing is so urgent that it should be addressed in the moment. Really, the only reason it seems important is because it is being considered now. Wait an hour and something else will come along that seems just as important. Wait another hour, and the pattern repeats. It's a fallacy. Nothing is as important as the thing you're thinking about in the present moment. Nothing. The key is to put time in the way of your actions.

When you make this a habit, you realize that most of the things that pop up are not that important at all. Not important enough to interrupt your thought processes, anyway.

I love to put time in the way of conversations with staff. In doing so, one of two things happens:

1. They figure it out for themselves.
    or
2. They realize it was never that important in the first place and they cancel the meeting.

The other thing that happens when you put time in the way is that they get a chance to prepare for the meeting with you. As one of my business coaches drilled into me, "If a meeting is worth having, it is worth preparing for."

For *every* meeting I have with any member of my team, I insist on an agenda ahead of time. I'll tell you exactly how it goes: they must email me a day before the meeting, and I ask them to consider the following:

1. What it is they specifically are having a problem with, or what the opportunity is
2. The three solutions that they are considering
3. Which solution they deem to be the one most likely
4. What questions they are going to ask me during the meeting

In my work with business owners, I insist on the same level of preparation for my coaching calls. Many times, I've refused to attend a call with a business owner unless they do this first.

Without this level of thought ahead of time, the meeting descends into a conversation about problems to which the business owner already knows the answer. Progress happens when you prepare and get to the conversation that you don't yet know exists. You do that by preparing in this way.

In reality, the meeting with your staff is only as good as its preparation. You could even say that all of the value in the meeting happens before the meeting. This is a standard you should refuse to let slip. The quality of the meeting and the outcomes will increase significantly when you adopt this approach.

What you'll also find is that the time they need from you decreases – but they feel like they're getting more. I am sure the open-door policy works for some business owners – mostly the ones in Hollywood movies – but I have yet to see how it works for anyone else who is serious about getting stuff done and freeing themselves from the day to day of the company.

3. Empathy

Empathy is the ability to put yourself in someone's shoes and be able to truly understand their situation and feelings. You're not born with empathy. It is learned. It is a skill that is developed over time through the study of books, of self, and through reflection on your day-to-day situations. But you're not born with it. Healthcare professionals usually have an abundance of compassion – but empathy does not come naturally to anyone.

Ironically, it's a skill that is honed by the deep study and implementation of marketing. Given that many healthcare professionals say that they don't like to market or that "it's not right to do so in healthcare," I find that quite remarkable. Perhaps they're just not able to put themselves in the shoes of a business owner who is trying to do his or her best for their patients and staff?

Seriously, you show me a great marketer and I'll show you someone who has empathy in abundance. I've learned over the last ten-plus years of leading people that this is one of the most important skills you can have.

The more that you can truly sit in the seat of your people, the more you begin to let go of the rigidness that often wrecks your company's growth.

Now what I mean by that is it is easy to have a fixed view of how you expect your employees to behave or act – or even how much effort or time they should give you. Over time, and particularly as you add more staff to your team, you learn that they all need be treated differently – it's the only way to be truly fair.

You have a greater ability to do that if you can better understand their thoughts and feelings. It stops you from taking some of the things they do, demand, ask for, or forget to do personally – as an attack on you – and instead helps you start to turn things around to see them from their point of view.

As an example, I was once adamant that I would need my employees to be able to start and finish at certain times that work for the company. Let's say 9 A.M. to 5 P.M. I had a rigid view of what I thought I needed in terms of availability to make the business successful.

As I've developed more empathy, I've come to realize that it's in *my* best interests to make sure that *their* best interests are also considered. That might be being able to collect children or finish early on certain days to do things that are important to them.

I can recall many instances where I have almost said or done something but stopped myself. Later, that turned out to be the best decision. That only happened because I put time in the way of making the decision and spent more time seeing the situation from someone else's point of view. Deploying empathy. As a CEO, you must quickly learn that sometimes what is best for the company is what is best for your best people. Empathy helps you get to that view.

4. Over-Communicate

If it is important enough to say once, you will have to say it 100 more times. Never get tired of saying the same thing over and over and certainly don't think that it is a bad thing. The genius of the great CEO is in finding different ways to say the same thing until it finally clicks with employees.

That could be big-picture information about the vision or latest strategy, or it could be more tactical in helping them understand how to implement the new script.

Understand that just because you said something once, that doesn't mean they understood it. It takes many chops of an axe for a big tree to fall. It isn't the final swing of the axe that causes the tree to fall – it's the 100 before the final one that made it possible. The CEO should never get tired of saying the same things – especially not if you're running your business by a set of guiding principles that you know to be true.

Principles never change, nor do they go out of date.

If you're running your business by tactics and fads, then you're always changing the scripts and your people will get easily confused. Politicians who chop and change their meaning to suit the day's news never get voted in. The ones who do are the ones who repeat and repeat again and again the meaning of their campaign and what they stand for.

In my practice, and in my coaching, I am always talking about the principles of business success and reminding my team of principles such as "people don't make quick decisions," "the fortune is in the follow up," "impulse decisions happen only if the price is under $100," and many more than I repeat almost daily.

But I never get bored of reminding my staff why these things are important.

In fact, I'd tell you that if your company ever goes through a revenue slump, it'll be because the principles have been lost or forgotten in favor of something new and exciting. Your job is to keep communicating the vision and never stop communicating the principles. This is not to be confused with telling a member of staff how to do his job every day. Anything more than showing someone three times how to do their job and you've likely tolerated everything that you're about to get from that person.

Remember: the first time it is your fault, the second it's theirs, and the third time is your fault for keeping them.

5. Help Them in Life

This is a huge one. I think that you need to be a very good life coach if you want to be a great CEO. There's no way you can just help your people with answering the phone or being better clinically and expect them to really improve.

The best people make the best employees. Said differently, if you can take the time to help someone find progress in their personal life, you usually get a very different person showing up for work the next day.

Another way to look at it is this: if you've got someone with serious issues happening at home that you choose to ignore, whatever you're asking them to do each day in your practice is really just going to go in one ear and out the other.

I believe you're better off spending 90 percent of your time with your employees making sure they're okay in their personal lives and 10 percent of it on their work. Most employees who don't perform well at work do so because they're a little lost in their home lives (and they're bringing that to work with them). I'm not saying that you can fix it or that all of them will even let you try, but I am saying that nine out of ten of them will appreciate the fact that you took an interest. And really, all they want is someone to listen to them in a non-judgmental manner. If you happen to have a suggestion or two to help them, that is a bonus.

Your people have got to leave your world as better people. That might be in their confidence, their ability to make better decisions, how seriously they take themselves, or how they view their capabilities. If they're not developing as people, they'll never develop as employees.

Okay, so we've come a long way in the last few chapters on recruiting and keeping A players. In the next chapter, we're going to look at what happens when they all come together. How people work together – especially when you're not around – is what defines your culture. Developing culture is another one of the top jobs of a CEO. Turn the page and let's look at how to make it happen.

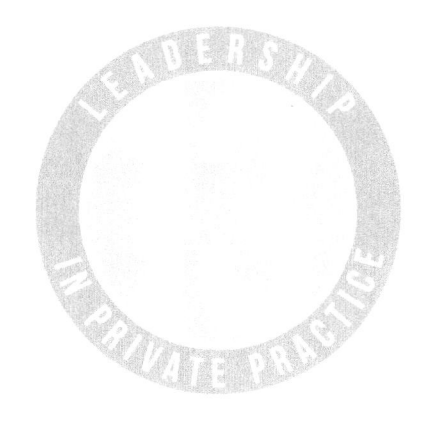

DEVELOPING A GREAT CULTURE

If cash is king, then culture is queen! And it seems that with the arrival of big tech companies such as Google and Facebook – and the movies that depict their supposedly amazing cultures – a lot of small businesses are trying to emulate what they're seeing. I think this is a mistake.

Casual stuff such as sleep pods, ping pong tables, ready-made breakfast stations, and allowing dogs into the office have been introduced into the workplace of many companies in an attempt to improve culture. The problem is they're not developing culture – they're giving staff perks. The two are very different.

I am sure it works well for some companies – especially the massive ones backed by venture capitalists, angel investors, or Wall Street. Basically, companies that are generally using someone else's money to pay their staff and give these types of perks.

But in the real world of small business – where all of the money we generate comes from our own creativity or labor – I think those things could lead to a culture of entitlement, making fun the focus of work rather than productivity and profit.

Perks are fine, but they also have nothing to do with culture. They're just a feature of a workplace that attracts a certain type of person. You're not instantly going to have a great culture *just* by letting your front desk girl bring her dog into work, or because you allowed your physical therapist to play your marketing assistant at ping pong when patients don't show up at the clinic.

WHAT IS CULTURE AND HOW DO YOU DEFINE A GOOD ONE?

Like leadership, culture is a concept and it is open to many different interpretations (hence so much confusion on these important topics). Some say it is how you treat each other. Others say it is how the staff behave when the boss isn't there. I agree with both of those. But this definition is the one that I really like: *the culture of your company teaches people how to behave*. New employees who arrive are instantly looking for clues on what is acceptable and what isn't at the company and they'll rise to or sink to the level that you accept. It's that simple.

Let's consider this all-too-frequent scenario that I am sure has happened to you before.

During the interview process, you find someone you think is your perfect candidate. They're attentive, punctual, and they say and do all of the right things in the interview to get them the job. They arrive for their first day on the job extra early and they stay late. They bring the coffees and snacks in for their new teammates and they're relentless with their questions, wanting to discover everything they can about the business.

This continues for the whole of the new employee's first week. The pattern stretches on into weeks three and four but then, all of a sudden, the employee starts to arrive on time (not early) and forgets to bring coffee.

They've also stopped asking questions of other staff members and one or two things are not getting done because he or she "didn't realize it was their job" (even though they've been doing it for the last three weeks).

Then, in week five, the person who used the same alarm clock to be fifteen minutes early for work – and drove the same way to work for the first four weeks – starts to be late.

All of a sudden, the "long line in Starbucks" is to blame for why they're "only one minute late."

The next week, he or she is repeatedly five minutes late and the excuse is that the "traffic is really bad."

By weeks seven and eight, there's a clear lack of engagement, deadlines are missed, time is spent gossiping, and lunchtime has turned into 45 minuets when in the first four weeks this person was never hungry. In the first four weeks, they told you they are "too busy for food' and they always worked through lunch.

In weeks seven and eight, they now eat so much food you worry you'll need to widen the doors or get them a bigger chair.

In weeks nine, ten, and eleven, it becomes apparent that this person has developed a love affair with the coffee machine. They're also on Facebook and Instagram so much that they need to bring their phone charger to work. You also begin to realize how "unlucky" this person is. They've bought six different alarm clocks and none of them work (causing them to be late every day).

And there's more! Their coat is always on five minutes before the end of the day and they're heading out the door with the car started and screeching out of the parking lot less than thirty seconds after their workday has ended.

It's funny that the same alarm that doesn't work in the morning always seems to alert them that it is time to leave – at the same five minutes early every day.

What went wrong?

How did this employee who could arrive early, who was engaged and wanted to learn so much that they'd stay behind after work end up sinking to such a poor standard? Simple. Culture caught up with him or her. That's what happened. Your culture – the one that you've created – taught this person what they could and couldn't get away with. The only thing this employee learned was what would or wouldn't be tolerated and she slowly adapted to the standards of the rest of the team. The culture of this company taught this new employee what is acceptable and normal. The culture was responsible for turning a good starter into a poor finisher.

Culture is really what you tolerate from your people.

That's why you've got to be so aware of the small things that you're going to tolerate in the company – particularly in the early years. It is much easier to shape culture than it is to change it.

Most businesses with a poor culture didn't consciously shape it that way. It just happened. It evolved. And it nearly always happened because of a lack of courage on the part of the leader.

Write this down or highlight this next sentence: *at the root of all failed cultures is a lack of leadership*. At the root of all failed leadership is a lack of courage. If you don't have the courage to call out your employees for arriving *bang on time* (remember, on time is really one traffic light missed from being late – early is on time), for asking them not to use their cell phones, or for getting ready to leave before the workday is done, you will get mediocrity at best.

As for things like in-fighting, gossiping, and cliques or silos that slowly develop between groups of employees, you simply cannot tolerate any of those things if you want a culture that thrives.

You've got to fight to get a great culture.

You're going to have to say things and do things that some of your employees are not going to like at first, especially if they've come from places or worked for bosses who tolerate lower standards. But this doesn't mean it's wrong to say or do any of it.

Your natural tendency is to want to constantly improve. To hit higher standards or at least aim for them. Your staff might not be inclined this way, but it doesn't mean that they won't come up some of the way with you. You have to make a commitment to *never* relenting on what you want or what you will tolerate. Much like a mother who is always cleaning up after her kids, see it as part of your job!

More: if you're wanting to improve your culture, you've got to look at whether or not your staff trust each other and respect each other as well as the common goal that you're trying to achieve. Is it something that they want to be involved with? Or are they just there to pick up a pay check?

You've also got to consider if the staff are trusting of *you*. If they don't trust you, you've got a big problem. What's the first sign that they don't trust you? They're constantly pushing back at your attempts to drive growth and change.

They can say that they don't like what you're doing, but they shouldn't be leading a revolt every time you want to raise the prices or change a script. It's a sure sign that they don't trust you.

I say to my staff all the time, "I don't need you to like it or agree that it is right – I just need you to say you'll be willing to give it a try." I provide all of the tools, training, and resources we need to make it work. If it still goes wrong, it's all on me.

COMPANY VALUES TELL YOUR STAFF HOW TO BEHAVE

If your vision or mission is what you want to achieve, your company's values tell your people how to behave along the way to reaching your target. These values are things such as accountability, calling it tight, growth and learning, or putting each other first. Values also dictate your culture and how your people develop.

I believe a successful businessperson should be measured not just by profits but also by the success enjoyed by the people of the business. What is happening in their careers? What is happening in their lives? How are they developing as people?

Don't just default to how many perks you give your people to determine how good of a boss you think you are. As I said earlier in this chapter, perks are not what defines your company culture. Sure, they're great for employees at the time, but they come closer to driving entitlement more than culture. Same with money. All of the money in the world won't fix a bad marriage. It won't change an unruly employee either.

Here's another way to look at culture.

Culture is what happens when the business owner is not there. Culture is how you treat each other and handle conflict. It is about measuring, accountability, focusing on solutions, leaving drama and opinions at the door, calling it tight, saying what needs to be said, being kind yet firm, acknowledging each other's contributions, and expressing appreciation.

The biggest issue with most cultures is that they are not consciously created. They are allowed to form by chance. That type of culture won't make the difference you're looking for, especially if you're wanting to step back from the day-to-day running of the practice. Culture and how your people behave are fundamental to the growth of your company. Remember this: talents got them the job – how they behave and embrace the values of the culture help them keep it. Most employees get fired because of a lousy attitude, not because they lack the skills to do the job. It is unlikely they all arrived with a lousy attitude. It is more likely that your culture allowed the lousy attitude to shine. And if that happened, it's nearly always because of a lack of clearly defined – and strongly enforced – values.

THE FOUR THINGS THAT DICTATE YOUR PRACTICE CULTURE

Over the years, I've discovered that there are really only four specific things under your control that give you a chance of a great culture. They are all in sync with each other. Each one leverages the impact of the others and all four must be in place for your culture to be where you want it.

1. Your Hiring Process: Seek A Players

We've just spent two chapters covering the importance of the CEO hiring A players – and keeping them. Culture is an extension, the long tail wind, of the hiring process. Your culture has to start with the hiring process. Most people are going to lose their jobs because they're not a fit culture-wise. Bad culture hires happen because the process didn't weed them out.

Often, when I'm asked about how to fix "bad employees," I tell the business owner that it's likely already too late – the recruitment process allowed the situation to happen.

It allowed a *potential* A player into the company, but one whose values likely weren't inspected closely enough for a match. As well as making sure you find the true A players, the process also needs to be robust enough to ensure you don't get duped. There are more A player impersonators out there than you'd think. You better make sure your process does the job of exposing them.

If your hiring process doesn't involve a significant and in-depth discussion about the behavior and standards you expect – and even the culture of the places that they've worked in the past – you will be lucky not to get duped.

Many of the interviewees I have really liked let themselves down at this point in the interview process. When I start to ask them about their previous teammates – specifically, what they liked or didn't like about them – they'll often be disrespectful or derogatory toward them. I've even had someone sit there and tell me all about their previous bosses and how big of jerks they *all* were.

I was sitting there and thinking about how that was interesting – but also that I was likely the next in line to join this illustrious list of jerks.

What is more, I can often find out how loyal people are by asking this simple question: "How much notice do you need to give your current employer?" If they say, "Well I am *supposed* to give three weeks, but I can leave them tomorrow if you want me to," they're telling you something about who they really are.

Of course, they want to impress you, but they're about to leave the company that has been paying their rent and bills for the last two years in a bind. I don't think that is a decent thing to do.

Again, I wonder how long it will be before I am getting left in the same bind by this person who doesn't seem to understand that notice periods are there to ensure that the company – and all of its employees – are not left compromised?

Now, if the person says, "I have a three-week notice and I plan to work it even if I lose this position," I know I have found my candidate and I'd happily wait six weeks for them if needed.

The questions you ask in this part of the interview process need to be cleverly worded and well thought out. They cannot be from a list of the "Top 10 Interview Questions" you Googled the night before the interview. You'll end up with a fraud who has prepared a set of stock answers doing exactly what you did – Googling interview questions the night before.

Remember that the person you've interviewing has likely done more interviews than you've held. They've likely had more interviews than hot dinners. In comparison, you're possibly doing it only once or twice per year. This gives *them* a serious upper hand. Never forget you're going up against professional interviewees. Don't arrive an unprofessional interviewer or you will get beat every time.

2. Onboarding

The next thing that is needed is a solid and robust onboarding process that gives this person a chance of being successful. The onboarding process is designed to introduce them to all of the things they're going to have to do to be successful in the role and *train* them on how to do it. It can last up to ten to twelve weeks. The longer, the better.

The key word is *training*. Training tells them how to do it. *Coaching* takes places after the onboarding is finished and this is where you help them do it better.

For example, let's say someone comes into your practice and his role is on the front desk. Of course, one of the jobs is to answer the phone. When he first comes into the practice, he knows how to pick up the phone, say hello, and even book an appointment. But he doesn't know how *your* practice does any of those things. You must surely have your own unique way of greeting new and returning customers that you've evolved over time to improve the chances of the patient converting? To get them to do it the way you want them to do it, you've got to train them. After a few weeks, they'll be doing it better (at least they should be).

Then, assuming they pass their ninety-day probation period, you're now going to continuously show them how to do the job better. They'll be taught different ways of addressing objections or how to engage with the patients to make them feel more comfortable and invested in your clinic.

The point is, there's a difference between coaching and training, but both are vital.

If you want an employee to have any chance of success, you've got to have a structured onboarding process that, over the course of twelve weeks, takes them through all of their major responsibilities.

What are these responsibilities? They're the ones you listed in the job ad. Your ad should have contained the role's top ten tasks that the person hired will handle each day or week. The people who applied thought they could do those tasks. It makes sense then, to train them during the onboarding process on the exact things that you said they would need to do, don't you think?

If you don't do this, you're guilty of abdicating the success of the role and expecting them to know how to do things – which never happens with any employee, no matter how good they are. I'd go so far as to say that *not* having an onboarding process is how you turn good employees for other people into bad employees for you.

Employees can't be successful in their roles if they're not trained.

If they're not trained, they'll mess up tasks. If they mess up tasks, you or other members of the team become annoyed. Things start to get heated, emotional, and irrational and it's not long before you have an employee who is defending himself by suggesting that everyone is picking on him when things go wrong.

In that moment, you've lost your culture and it's difficult to regain until they leave. It's certainly on pause until they do.

EMPLOYEE WELCOME BOXES

The onboarding process in my businesses actually starts the day someone accepts the job. We've developed a "box of stuff" – better known as a "Welcome to the Company" box – that has, well, everything they're going to need to go through in the coming weeks as part of their onboarding. They get books I've written, testimonials from other clients and staff, and their own manual – specific to their role – to work through in the weeks ahead. They can literally see into the future and know what they're going to be learning in the next three months.

It works in schools, why not in business?

They also get a copy of our mission statement, core values, and company history, as well as a copy of our most recent three-day annual planning meeting notes. We want them to start their onboarding the right way and to know the company's back story.

Doing this also does a very good job of putting off the wrong people. When we give them their welcome box, they can see how diligent and thorough we are. They know they're coming to a company that is serious about training, coaching, results, and accountability. If they arrive for their first day after going through their welcome box, that is a good sign. If they *don't*, that's great too.

3. Reviews/Scorecards

Each individual member of the team must have their own scorecard – and a regular conversation supporting it. This comes in the form of a weekly or biweekly twenty- to thirty-minute review conversation with their manager or a senior person in the company. Depending on the size of the company, it could still be with you. Who conducts the meeting doesn't matter as much as it being done, and done without fail.

To say that I underestimated the role of the regular review process is an understatement. To be honest, I wasn't even good at doing annual reviews, never mind a weekly one. Why? Well, I simply didn't know what to do or say in them.

Plus, I always thought it would give the employee an excuse to ask for a pay raise – so I tended to try and avoid it. I'm serious. I was never a fan of doing them. However, since I've implemented employee reviews that happen every other week, I can tell you it is transformational for your culture and your team's performance.

GET YOUR FREE RESOURCE KIT: PAULGOUGH.COM/LEADERSHIP-RESOURCE

You are "shortening the feedback loop" on giving praise, on finding out what their issues are (at home or at work), and, quite candidly, giving them a kick in the ass!

Seriously, one of the questions we ask the team in our reviews is, "Where do you think you need a kick up the arse?" Notice the specific wording: where do *they* think they need a kick? I'm not *telling* them. I'm *asking* them. I'm asking them to be self-aware and take ownership, as well as suggesting that there's always room for improvement. What's more, I'm telling them that we're willing to help them do it.

Do I actually kick them up the arse? Literally, no. Figuratively, yes. This is tough love (one of our core values). Would I let my kids go through life underachieving or always letting themselves down? Of course not. I'm paying attention to that and I'm jumping in to give them a "kick up the arse" when I think they need it.

They might not like it at the time, but I know they will thank me later.

And even if they don't, it's *still the right thing to do*. That is my job as their father.

It is the same in the office. I'm willing to be disliked if it means ensuring my staff achieve their potential. I meant it when I once told an employee of mine that rather than see me as someone who is always on his back, he should be very grateful to have someone in his life who cares enough to want *him* to be better.

The review process is really just about making sure that someone on your team has their finger on the pulse of what's happening with employees.

The scorecards are there to keep the conversation objective. There should be some discussion about how the employee is feeling or what is happening in their lives – that is very important and should be encouraged.

However, it can't be at the expense of a conversation about the results they've achieved.

Never forget this: if the conversation is always about emotional stuff — drama — the job is too big for the employee and it's time to switch them out.

You need to be talking about the pre-identified objective measures. They are what determines the success this person will have in their role. What customer satisfaction score is this employee achieving? What is the lead conversion ratio the front desk is getting? What is the clinical outcome the PT is getting? What is their patient visit average ratio and why is it lower than everyone else on your team?

This is about you pointing out that the standards you need — that both of you agreed upon in the recruitment process — are not being hit. Said differently, with their current level of performance, they're not able to call themselves successful in the role.

Your reason for the review is to make sure that they're always striving toward higher standards and never allowed to dip for so long that it becomes a habit.

We all have days and perhaps weeks of not being on our game, but we can't tolerate it happening for months on end. That will bring your business down and it'll hurt your bottom line. Holding mini reviews frequently gives your employees a chance to get things off their chests, come up with ideas or spot opportunities, and feel valued as part of the team (all things we spoke about in Chapter 11 when we discussed retaining A players).

If they're having issues with other employees, this can come up in the conversation too. And when you do the review with the employee in question, you can approach the issue in a way that can bring both of them together, helping to maintain the health of your culture.

Seriously, scorecard reviews rock. Don't overlook them because you think you're too busy. If that is the current case, chances are you're too busy to do them because you're doing things you don't need to or shouldn't be doing – those would be spotted in the review.

4. Personal Development

Your people should always express a fondness for your company as being the place they discovered how to get more from themselves. It could be the place they learn to confidently sell, overcome fears and negative attitudes, and become involved in personal development. Of course, not everyone wants to do this, but the best ones really do.

Your team members should be learning how to handle rejection and disappointment. They should be learning basic success habits like punctuality, goal setting, and time management. They should be developing an interest in learning outside of the workplace to simultaneously improve their performance at work. They should be developing their work ethic and a love of learning as well as improving their communication skills, persuasive ability, motivation, and knowledge about people.

When your employees are transformed like this or are involved in a process that is continuously transforming who they are and who they think of themselves as being, this is when you achieve a culture you can celebrate.

Of course, they don't all want to take part in it. They don't all want to learn everything they can while they're with you. However, the opportunity to do so must be there and there must be a list of poster boys or girls who are products of your system's success.

You might think all of this is how the employees should arrive anyway. Big mistake. I learned this one the hard way. School mostly sets them up to memorize information and rewards them with a PhD in something that is mostly irrelevant. As for society, it mostly sets people up to underachieve with the entitlement culture that has been created by the government. Apathy is a very addictive drug and the government loves to dispense it to anyone who wants a daily dose.

After a few years of running a practice, I realized that I had a choice.

I could *expect* that my people would show up the perfect finished product (thus contributing to the entitlement culture) or I could expect nothing and instead give people an opportunity to become the best versions of themselves through my culture.

When you have your team talking about what books they're reading and what podcasts they're listening to, or asking you what else or who else they can learn from about topics related to personal development, you know you are on a rocket ship to the moon and your team is driving it.

Contrary to that, if you have a team of people who only want to talk about what they're watching on TV or gossiping about who is doing what or buying what, you are unlikely to get where you want to be.

I'm not saying I've cracked the code on personal development, but I know I lead by example. In doing so, I inspire the inspirable.

If my recruitment process is set up to look for candidates who have an interest in developing as people, then I have a chance of it happening. And, in doing so, I have a chance that my culture will be one of high performance instead of high maintenance. After all, the difference between effort and struggle is negative emotion. A commitment to personal development is about turning a struggle into a challenge. When that challenge is overcome, accomplishment is the reward.

Overlook personal development in your practice at your own peril. In today's competitive marketplace, your only leverage is your people. Not your clinical skills. It really does pay to create a culture that inspires people to develop themselves.

As always, it starts with *you*. You show me a business owner who stopped developing when he or she left school and I'll show you a crappy culture.

Okay, so let's move on from people and culture. In the next chapter, we're going to bring everything together and determine the highest-value work you can do. We will talk about the two things that the most successful CEOs have in common. Come with me and I'll share the secret.

AVOID THE NUMBER ONE REASON BUSINESSES FAIL

At this point, I bet you're thinking something like, *It's okay for this guy. He sounds like he's got this whole leadership in private practice thing taken care of...* as if I've got a handle on *everything* in my practice? That I'm sitting on the beach here in Florida, in between dropping my kids off at school and hanging out in Starbucks, checking my online banking app, counting all the cash that comes in, and making a phone call or two when there's not as much in there as I would like?

Well, that's not quite true.

There are no beaches in Orlando, and I don't care too much for Starbucks.

No, seriously, that's not how it works. I might have "written the book" on leadership, but that doesn't mean that I've cracked the code. I am not sure that is ever possible. I am a permanent work in progress. My office is a construction site and the building will never be complete. Every day is a school day and as long as I am growing a company, I will need to be growing my ability to get a handle on the challenges presented by growth.

I accept the responsibility and the reward will be more hills to climb.

The irony of business success is that your reward for growth – and overcoming challenges – is new challenges that seem to get bigger and more daunting each time you push through to the next level. Yippee!

As I said way back in Chapter 1, if you knew then what you know now, you'd never have started your own business. But you have, and the best thing you can do now is commit to being successful at it. Go big or go home.

What I've outlined in this book is what I know now based upon the tests that business and life have thrown at me thus far. Like I said at the start, this is a field report. It's based upon the lessons I've learned and tools I've picked up to this point.

Yet, the marketplace is always changing. The environment and conditions are constantly evolving. Business leaders need to be able to adapt with those changing circumstances and not resist them just because they don't want to have to learn or do something new.

I wrote this book while simultaneously living through and running my businesses in the midst of the COVID-19 pandemic. It threw up economic and financial chaos – not to mention public fear – on a scale that was unprecedented. I had to adapt on what seemed like a daily basis. Business hurled new, unexpected challenges at me at a rate I'd never known in more than a decade of being in business. A week become the new month. A month the new quarter. It was fluid, to say the least.

But the truth is, I relished the whole situation.

Although I didn't want any of it to be happening, and I'd rather it hadn't, it did. And you're always better off living in the "is" world than the "I wish it wasn't" world.

Throughout the pandemic, I chose to embrace the events that were being tossed at me. I was taking tests and then quickly learning lessons. It was nothing like what I was taught at school, that's for sure. It forced me to learn about myself and evaluate my skills against the needs of my company. The situation allowed me to reflect on what I needed to do to improve and keep pushing through, turning the mess into an opportunity to come out the other side even stronger. Isn't that what business leaders do? Make things happen even when all of the odds are stacked against us?

BEWARE THE COMFORTABLE PILLOW OF SUCCESS

As a kid, I was good at sports. Always first on the team for anything to do with pretty much any sport at school. And the problem was, *I was good at any sport*. Seriously, that was the problem! I could turn my hand to anything and expect to be good at it. So good that I remember my dad warned me at a young age that being successful brings with it a curse. The curse is that you can easily take success for granted. Just because you've been successful once, you think you can easily repeat it without having to do the work.

His exact words were, "It's very easy to fall asleep on the comfortable pillow of success." He cautioned me against thinking that I was always going to be successful just because I was successful once. I think that conversation has stuck with me throughout my business life and it's served me very well.

GET YOUR FREE RESOURCE KIT: PAULGOUGH.COM/LEADERSHIP-RESOURCE

Privately, I think I'm anxious that I'll one day fall asleep at the helm of my business.

That motivates the heck out of me.

I don't really want the trappings of business success – flashy cars, big houses, expensive clothes or watches – and I don't even care if people know I am successful. I just want the feeling of accomplishment that comes with success. It's a drug to me. I want to be successful just because there's an opportunity to do so. It's a way of living – not a thing you buy.

Equally, I want to do the work just because there's work to do be done and I'll feel accomplishment when it's done. The beer in my local tavern always tastes better when the work is done.

As a result, I am constantly looking for deeper insight into something I already know a lot about. It could be a new relevance or meaning of managing people that I'm looking for, a new understanding of key ratios, or information on how to recruit even better people for my company. That's why I am always learning.

To me, that's the joy of being in business.

That's the *real* reward.

Business ownership gives you a chance to learn something new – even if it's about something old – and you get to discover more about yourself that you never would have learned had you not been in business. Isn't that what life is all about? Isn't that what we're all searching for? What if the purpose of life really is to grow as much as you can and realize your full potential?

Kids come out of school each day with smiles on their faces and those smiles usually get bigger as they tell their parents exactly what they learned that day. Look closely and you'll see *real joy*. I see it on the faces of my kids every day given the age they're at right now. The simplest thing they're learned is enough to make their day (and subsequently mine).

Imagine if you left school and you spent your whole life never again experiencing that type of joy. Making money makes you happy. At best, it is a moment in time of pleasure. Now learning and growing, that brings fulfillment. And fulfillment is a drug that lasts must longer than pleasure. If in doubt, focus on fulfillment. It'll make you very happy and the pleasure that comes is easier to savor.

People in the business community talk about wanting to make an impact. I'm sure that's true. But more than anything, I think business owners are searching for relevance and purpose. Business offers you the opportunity for both. If you do it right, you get both in abundance and your impact increases as a happy by-product.

Sure, business ownership can bring pressure and, with it, its fair share of frustrations. But I think the pressure is a privilege. It reminds me that I am in a position that is relevant and that my life has meaning. If I'm frustrated or angsty, it's just a sign that I'm taking a test for which I need to better prepare.

And being in business does present you with tests.

Whatever the tests in life, multiply them by ten when you run a business and add in all of the variables that come with owning a company. The tests *are* challenging, but they really just test your resolve and help develop your character.

In fact, they reveal your character.

"Who you're becoming along the way" (as you grow your company) is an important thing for you to consider. Many don't. Most just think about how much money they're making or how much power it brings them.

GET YOUR FREE RESOURCE KIT: PAULGOUGH.COM/LEADERSHIP-RESOURCE

They talk about the journey being more important than the destination. And I happen to believe that's true. That's because, as entrepreneurs, we never actually arrive at the destination. We always kick it down the road. We get close to the destination and then we realize we want a new one that is always bigger and better. We were once happy with $500,000, but now that we are getting close to it, we decide we want $1,000,000. In that respect, it has to be about the journey. And besides, what would you do when you reach the destination?

Retire?

Heck no!

If you're anything like me, I couldn't think of anything worse than sitting on a beach for weeks or months on end, absent of a purpose or a reason to learn and grow.

Retirement is one of those things that you want to be able to fall back on only if your body won't let you do what you really want to do. Life is about having a sense of achievement, pursuing personal growth and ambition for your *whole* life – not just some of it. Why would I want to give any of those things up?

Ever wondered why basketball or soccer coaches carry on well into their seventies? It's not because they need the money. And even after they step down from coaching, they still want some role with one of their previous teams, maybe on the board or as ambassador. They do so because they want the sense of purpose and achievement that they've become addicted to. They discovered it along the way to mastering their craft. That's what business gives us the opportunity to do – and, in that respect, I do think that all of the challenges it presents us with are happening *for* us, not *to* us.

STRETCH YOUR CAPACITY THRESHOLD

Being a business owner stretches your capacity threshold – your ability to deal with multiple things happening around you all at once. It forces you to manage things simultaneously when most people think and act sequentially. That is, most people do the next thing when they finish the last thing. Sounds logical, right? And it is. But not to you and me. That sounds like it's too sensible and boring. And slow. We would never get the business off the ground or grow it if we thought that way. You and I have to think simultaneously if we want to build a business.

We have start the hiring process for one job while simultaneously onboarding the latest recruit who just started last week, manage cash flow, coach the team, look after the marketing plan and talk to the landlord about getting another room in the building just in case business continues to trend up. If we thought sequentially – like they teach at school – we'd never get anything done.

You also have to look after more than just yourself.

Looking after yourself and your own family is one thing. But doing that *and* taking care of dozens of other families (of the people you employ) and ensuring they can all meet their rent is another obligation altogether. If you can't make payroll, they can't make rent. In the end, the responsibility stops with you.

It takes a special kind of person to be able to accept that type of burden. It needs to be experienced to understand just how big the responsibility really is. It is certainly misunderstood by those in the media who claim that business owners are "greedy" or, worse, those pesky politicians (who have never run a business or risked their own money) who seem to think that business ownership has nothing but an upside and that we should pay more and more in taxes as a result.

Through the coronavirus outbreak, I had the responsibility of leading my companies through the biggest crisis I am ever likely to live through – and at the same time make my family feel safe and protected. I'd worked so hard to build a wonderful lifestyle for my family that I wasn't prepared to let even the excuse of coronavirus come up in the conversation about how it might affect us. Not once was it affecting us ever considered an option.

If ever there was a period in my life that I was grateful for having invested in business training and coaching, it was throughout COVID-19.

I had to juggle thinking about my business and my employees, not to mention taking care of clients, with making sure that the biggest crisis in modern times was never felt in my home. I was only able to do so because of the skills I've learned along the way and because I choose to see life and the obstacles it throws at me as opportunities to learn about myself. It's a mindset, an outlook, that I've honed over the years on my journey toward building a better business and a better life.

You can't really separate the person from the business. The two are interwoven. But one is more responsible than the other for success or failure. The business never lets the person down. **But the person nearly always lets the business down**. *That is the real root cause of why businesses fail.* It's that the person running the business simply isn't equipped to do so at the level the business requires. This is what you must avoid. Don't become an owner being run by a business.

"WORKING ON YOURSELF" – NOT JUST ON THE BUSINESS

I believe a CEO must be constantly working on himself, not just on the business. It's too easy to say, "I work on the business." If you do, that's great! Author Michael Gerber made that phrase famous in the book *The E Myth*. But I think that's a waste of time if you're not working on the most important part of the business – **you.**

How can the business ever improve if you don't?

Your business will never outgrow your own development as you're the one driving that growth. When you stop learning about business, it stops growing.

Candidly, I will often say that "I am the business."

That's because no matter how big the business gets, or how many employees come into the business, in the end, when all is said and done, I am still the business.

Sure, I've had the help of a lot of great people. But ask yourself how they got there. I recruited the people in the first place. And yes, I've got great customers in all of my businesses. But how did they get there? I built the sales systems to get the customers.

I created the culture. I understood the finance and executed on what the numbers showed me. That's why I say that "I am the business." It's not arrogance or ignorance – it's fact. It is also why I never worry about the business. I only ever worry that I am working on myself enough to keep up with the needs of the business. Big difference.

I remember when COVID-19 first started rearing its ugly head. Physical therapy businesses were hit hard because, understandably, people were frightened about human-to-human contact and the risk of the virus spreading. It caused my own practice to close completely and, by the same turn of events, it also exposed the consultancy business that focuses on helping private practice owners like you.

At the time, practices were closing down on a daily basis. During a phone call with my mother, she asked me if I had any concerns about the virus as it pertained to my business.

When she asked me, I responded abruptly, "Why would I?"

I went on to tell her what I just told you. That "I am the business." Sure, I might lose some revenue, but I will not lose my business because "I am the business." I am the one with the business skills that built the business in the first place. As long as coronavirus doesn't take those skills from me, I am not worried one bit.

There's a level of confidence that comes from developing your business skills. Show me a clinic owner frightened for the future and I'll show you one absent of the skills needed to run the business, who is unable to adapt to the changing marketplace.

There's a reason that 96 percent of businesses go bust every ten years. It's because, historically, the marketplace – the conditions and the environment – change every ten years.

Ever notice how a financial contraction – or a recession, as it is often known – seems to happen every ten years or so? Well, it also seems to wipe out most businesses each time it does and that's why most businesses never make it to celebrate their tenth birthday.

But it isn't the economy that causes them to go bust – someone in their industry survives and makes more. It's because the business owner isn't equipped to weather the storm. They lack the skills. It's easy to make money when there's money flowing. But, and as Warren Buffett says, when the tide goes out you get to see who has been swimming naked. Basically, you get to see who has been making a living absent of real business skills.

Never underestimate the power that you get from working on yourself.

Rather than thinking it's always about getting a "better business," my tip is to think of it in terms of becoming a *better you*. Inevitably, what follows is a better business.

If there's one single thing that I hope you take from this book, it's the idea that to be a great CEO who runs a successful practice, you must be obsessed with *becoming* better at it. It's an action that is required. It's not a thing that you ever achieve. No, you're constantly in pursuit of it, knowing that, at every point, if you are becoming better, the goal post is moving and it's moving because you're getting better at making it move. But at the same time, the number of life choices is increasing. And remember, like I said many times in the book, the people with the best lives have the best choices.

If the destination changed, it was your choice to change it. If you started off thinking you'd be happy with $150,000 per year and now you want $250,000 per year, that's your choice. You earned the right to that because of the skills you've added.

If you thought you wanted just enough profit to cover a jacuzzi in the garden, but now you want fifty-foot swimming pool and a slide thrown in for the kids to shoot down every day before school, that's your choice. You earned the right to it.

If you started off thinking that you would be happy with two weeks' vacation every year, but now you're wanting to take three months to travel round Europe each summer, that's your choice. You earned the right to it. Don't let anyone suppress you when it comes to what you want and rightfully deserve as a result of your business success.

If you want a new yacht, go get it! Just invite your staff out on it from time to time.

If you want the third car – a Ferrari, just to drive to and from church in style – go get it! If you want to give it all to the kids, do it! It's your choice. You earned it. You did the hard yards.

And like I said earlier in the book, you'll always be rewarded in public for the work you do in private. However you choose to live or spend the fruits of your labor, that is on you. Screw anyone who doesn't like how you're spending your hard work. Seriously, tell them their opinion isn't necessary. The truth is they're just in awe of the fact that someone can focus for so long on something and actually see something through to producing enough value that people want to pay you handsomely for it.

Whatever stage of business ownership you're at, there's a great journey that awaits. Never underestimate the advantages that having a more successful business can give you – or just what it takes to get to that point. The road to business success is lonely. It's frustrating and you'll likely isolate yourself from many people you knew when you first started.

But, it's well worth it.

I can tell you from firsthand experience, the juice is definitely worth the squeeze.

The journey justifies the means.

The reward is worth the risk.

I've loved every moment of the journey that I've been on to get to this point in my life. I'm very happy, I'm fulfilled in many areas of my life and I am who I am because of many of the things that I've been forced to learn about myself through my business building journey. For that I am delighted I chose to start a company.

You've started.

You're here now doing it.

My tip is to find ways to enjoy it and give it your best shot. Don't get to the other end and regret that you didn't become the business owner – or the person – who you could have been. And never forget that if your goal is a very successful business, it requires a very skilled business owner. However you slice the pie, in the end, it all comes down to the relentless pursuit of advancing your business skills.

YOUR NEXT STEPS TO BECOMING A BETTER CEO

Before we finish the book together, and assuming you like what you've read, I'd like to quickly tell you about other ways I can help you continue to develop your business skills. And, give your access to the type of business coaching that can help you grow your business – and enhance your lifestyle – beyond where it is today.

If you learned something from me that you want to explore further, or I've sparked your interest in wanting to take your business skills to the next level, there are a few ways we can work together now that this book is almost over. Here they are:

1. **The Ultimate CEO Toolkit, an instant-access binder with everything you need to do your job successfully**
2. **Business Success Coaching Programs for various levels**
3. **CEO Mastermind Program (application only)**

1. THE ULTIMATE CEO TOOLKIT

The Ultimate CEO Toolkit contains all of the essential resources, templates, and checklists that every CEO needs to do their job correctly.

In short, it stops you from "winging it" or making it up as you go along. It is a "briefcase" loaded with everything that you'll need to get focused, manage your team, create the marketing plan, manage the cash, hire your people, onboard them correctly, and develop the culture. It includes (but is not limited to):

- **Every job ad** for every position in your practice (therapist, office manager, marketing assistant, front desk, salesperson, etc.)
- **Detailed scorecard** for every position in your company
- **12-week onboarding process** for every position in your practice
- **Scorecard conversation** templates (for performance reviews)
- **12-month marketing plan** templates
- **Scripts for every sales situation in your practice** (a sales playbook)
- **Strategic planning meeting templates** and checklists
- **Annual planning meeting** templates and accompanying checklists
- **Examples of weekly, monthly, and quarterly meeting** conversations (structure and follow-up rhythm)
- **Finance tools** (plug-and-play cash flow forecast and profit and loss templates – just enter your numbers and watch it all come to life)
- **Annual budget templates**
- Plug-and-play **staff performance dashboards**
- *And so much more – including many of the things you've read about in this book!*

GET YOUR FREE RESOURCE KIT: PAULGOUGH.COM/LEADERSHIP-RESOURCE

The Ultimate CEO Toolkit is a treasure chest full of tools and templates that will save you years in trying to create yourself. It'll short cut the process of getting a handle on doing your job at the highest possible level, leaving you free to think strategically and adding value to your company.

For example, you won't have to write the job ads that often hold you back from hiring more quickly than you should – I've pre-written all of them for you.

When you do hire someone, you'll have a clear and precise onboarding pathway for every employee to give them the best chance of being successful.

You'll also know precisely how to performance manage your staff with check-in conversations that reflect their scorecards.

You'll also get a sales playbook to give to your front desk team to make sure they're able to do their job (with converting patients) as well as marketing plan templates to support your growth.

Basically, you're getting pre-written templates and resources that I've developed over the last ten-plus years of building my companies and you can have them instantly.

You get instant digital access to everything and can download it right away.

Plus, after you place your order, I'll send you a physical "briefcase" full of all the things I've mentioned above that can sit on your desk in your office to pull from as you need. I'll also comb through my hard drives and office looking for anything else that I use to manage my businesses that I think will come in handy and include it for you. Look out for a few pleasant surprises.

TO GET THE ULTIMATE CEO TOOLKIT, HEAD OVER TO:

www.paulgough.com/ceo-toolkit

2. BUSINESS SUCCESS COACHING PROGRAMS

What is business coaching? Perhaps you've been involved in it in the past, perhaps not? To me, it is the most valuable thing that anyone who has "business owner" in their title can ever invest in. If you've enjoyed this book, it shouldn't be lost on you how I came to be able to write it. I could not have written this book were it not for the business coaching I've had over the years.

No one can build a successful business, past where they are now, without a second voice in the conversation. To me, that's the real value of coaching. It's as simple as this: if you knew the answers, you'd have solved the problem already. If you knew what your business was needing to get to the next level, you'd have done it by now.

The best person to come up with an idea for your business is you, but you also need someone to question what you're thinking to ensure that what you're about to do is the right thing and won't lead to other often-unforeseen challenges.

What is more, you always want to make sure that what you're working on is the right thing at the right time. It is possible to work on the right thing at the wrong time and, sadly, this is the downfall of many a business owner. They are what I referred to in this book as "busy fools". Always doing something – but never achieving anything.

If you can see the value in having a conversation with someone who points out your blind spots, offers insights, and poses questions that stimulate higher-level conversations about your business and how you should best use your time, you will love the business coaching I can offer you.

We've been working with private practice owners like you for many years – helping them navigate the different phases of business growth as well as the challenges that growth brings.

Whether the challenge is marketing, managing people, culture, finance, or scale, I've passed through every phase of business ownership and been able to remove myself from a business and still make a profit. The latter is something that makes me very uniquely qualified to coach you on as very few in private practice ever achieve it.

At this point, I am familiar with almost every challenge or obstacle that you're likely to be dealing with in your practice. That's how I can confidently tell you that my coaching services can help you.

What is more, we can often spot your challenge in minutes.

Right now, something is holding you back – and you're unlikely to be able to work out what it is on your own simply because you're too close to the business; you're likely to be lost in your own head. And that is a very common thing to happen to a business owner and it's easy to stay there. That is because you can't solve problems with the level of thinking that gets you into the problems in the first place. That is why you need a second voice in your conversations so that you can change your thinking so that you change your actions and ultimately your results. That is what coaching does. That's why it's vital to your sustained success.

You might have been stuck for a year – but it's highly possible that we can find the reason why in a matter of minutes. It's nearly always quite obvious to the person who is not emotionally attached to the business. That's where having a business coach and being around a peer group can help – they speed up the journey to success.

I've been working with clinic owners for many years and have created a coaching company that is multi-level – meaning I can help you at any phase of business.

We can help the fledgling practice owner finally find momentum and bring in new patients consistently, and we're able to help the practice owner who is trying desperately hard – often too hard – to get past the point of the business being too heavily reliant upon their day-to-day involvement.

If you've been in business for more than two years and you're stuck at the same level, we can help you get moving again.

If you've started, but you're not going as fast as you would like, we can help you accelerate your growth.

We can help you with marketing, recruitment decisions, understanding your numbers, financial literacy, speeding up your decision making, and, above all, making the best decisions about your business and eventually removing yourself from it (if that's what you want).

We'll also share with you what we're learning from working with other our successful business owner clients so that you can learn from them. You can find out how you match up to other practices of your size and type. Are you more or less profitable? Are you working longer hours than they are? What opportunities are they maximizing that you might not be? We can share all of our insights to help you get to the next level faster. We've created an amazing community and there's real power (and leverage) in being able to access a community of like-minded practice owners.

IF YOU WANT TO KNOW MORE, JUST GO TO THE SITE BELOW AND FILL OUT THE FORM:

www.paulgough.com/coaching

(You can also send an email to paul@paulgough.com with the subject line "Coaching.")

After you reach out, a member of my coaching team will be in touch to find out what you're looking for, explain the different levels of coaching we offer, and help determine which is appropriate for you and your growth goals.

We work with practice owners across the US, Canada, the UK, and Europe, as well as places including Thailand, Dubai, Australia, New Zealand, and Brunei. Basically, wherever you are in the world, we can help you. With modern technology and the Internet, it's never been easier.

3. CEO MASTERMIND PROGRAM

The third way we can work together is via my exclusive CEO Mastermind Program. This is my highest-level coaching program and it is by application only. It's only for those who are wanting to grow their business and simultaneously remove themselves from it.

Some practice owners are addicted to being involved in their business every day and at every level. They love being in the treatment room all day long and don't want to give that up. This program is *not* for that person.

But there's a new and growing breed of private practice owners who recognize that the biggest reward – in terms of both finance and lifestyle – comes from being at the CEO level of the business where you are running the business but removed from day-to-day involvement. Put another way, you own the trains but you don't drive them.

If you are one of those practice owners, you will love this program.

In the CEO Mastermind Program, all of the conversations are about recruiting the right people, building an organizational chart with the right structure, understanding the numbers, investing the profits, and making plans for future growth.

The program is designed to move you from sitting down every day and thinking about what work _you_ need to do – and instead thinking about _who_ needs to do it for you. That's when you shift from operator to CEO.

It's about moving you from thinking about your relationship with your patients as being the most important thing – to realizing that the most important relationship is the one you have with your team (and letting your team build relationships with your patients). That's when you shift from operator to CEO.

If you're ready to shift from operator to CEO and finally remove yourself from the day-to-day running of the business, this is the program for you.

And to my knowledge, it is the only program that exists that is exclusively about *getting you out of the day-to-day grind of your practice.*

When you join CEO Mastermind Program, you're getting access to the ultimate peer group. It's nine other business owners with the same aspirations as you – with many possibly already doing what you want to be able to do, having already removed themselves from the practice, yet still making more money.

It is like having your own board of directors, something that every successful business needs. It's an opportunity to ask questions of very smart business owners.

The primary function of the CEO Mastermind Program is to provide you, the business owner, with the knowledge, insights, perspective, and distinctions – not to mention accountability – required to reduce bad decisions, increase good decisions, and execute consistently on the right things in your business.

Beyond that, a board serves to help you identify and eliminate risk.

If you can get advice from people who are just a few decisions ahead of you, or who have made the mistakes already, you're instantly ahead.

If you can get your plan or latest idea stress-tested by a board of ten (including me) who are completely emotionally removed and independent of any bias toward the outcome (and even your feelings), you're going to be sure that what you're about to do is the right thing. This allows you to go back to your practice and execute on the next steps to get to where you want to be, knowing it's the right use of your time.

We meet four times per year in groups of ten. This program is available by application only. **Send an email to paul@paulgough.com to find out if it's a good fit for you** and for more information on how to apply to the CEO Mastermind Program when a space becomes available.

So there you go! Those are the next steps that are available to you to continue to develop your business skills with me. Choose which one works for you and I'll look forward to working with you more closely. That's also a wrap for another book (you can find my others at www.paulgough.com/books).

I hope you've enjoyed reading this book as much as I have enjoyed writing it.

I wish you all the good fortune in the world as you continue on your journey to building a business that makes you proud. In that respect, and even though we don't know each other, we're kindred spirits.

If this book has inspired you or given you some hope for a better future for your business, it will have been worth every second that I've invested in writing it and all of the lessons that I've had to learn to be able to be in a position to do so.

I write all of my books with the goal of motivating and inspiring lasting success, and I do that by sharing real lessons of tests that I've taken in my life and in my businesses. If I can help you avoid one mistake or setback, or, help you to take an opportunity that you would have missed, I will have achieved my goal.

If you've benefitted from this book, I'd love to hear about how it has impacted both you and your business. Please feel to reach out to me at paul@paulgough.com with your thoughts. It would also mean the world to me if you would tell another private practice owner about this book.

Finally, well done for getting to this point in the book. It says a lot about you and your commitment to yourself and your business. I'm impressed.

To your success,
Paul Gough
www.paulgough.com/books
paul@paulgough.com
Tel: (US) 407 567 0086

ABOUT THE AUTHOR

PAUL GOUGH is the No.1 bestselling author of "The New Patient Accelerator Method", "The Physical Therapy Hiring Solution", and "To Sell is Healthy", three revolutionary books on marketing, hiring and sales for physical therapists. He's also an international speaker and a former professional soccer physical therapist turned successful clinic owner from the UK. Paul is the founder of the Paul Gough Physio Rooms – a successful four location cash pay clinic that he started from a spare room in his home whilst having had no money and no business or marketing skills. Paul has since scaled his clinic from zero to $1+, and what's most impressive is that he's done all of that in a country with a completely free, "socialist" health care system (one that provides physical therapist services for FREE for all UK residents) as his main competitor.

He is a true small business success story; he is now the owner of five companies, all of which are in three different markets and in two different countries – two of those companies have achieved million dollar+ revenues.

Paul is the host of the top-rated podcast "The Paul Gough Audio Experience: Business Lessons For Physical Therapists" (available on iTunes, Soundcloud, Spotify, Anchor and Stitcher). He is also a "Small Business ICON" WINNER in 2016, an award that is selected from all across Infusionsoft's 45,000+ global customers.

He is widely regarded, both in America and around the world, as a leading authority on direct to consumer marketing, and he has a proven track record of helping physical therapists attract cash pay patients, growing their practices, increasing profits, freeing up their time, and radically shifting their entrepreneurial thinking.

GET YOUR FREE RESOURCE KIT: PAULGOUGH.COM/LEADERSHIP-RESOURCE

ALSO BY PAUL GOUGH:

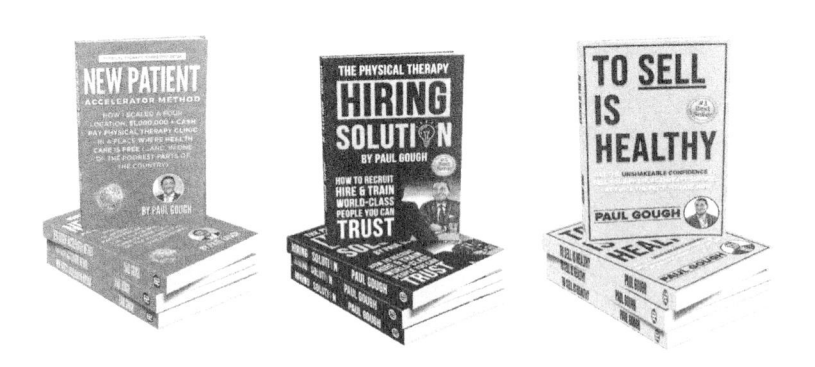

New Patient Accelerator Method:
"How I Scaled a Four Location, $1,000,000 + Cash Pay Physical Therapy Clinic - In a Place Where Health Care Is Free (...And, in One of the Poorest Areas of the Country)"
www.PaulsMarketingBook.com

The Physical Therapy Hiring Solution:
"How to Recruit, Hire and Train World-Class People You Can Trust"
www.PaulsHiringBook.com

To Sell Is Healthy:
"Get The Unshakeable Confidence to Sell Your Physical Therapy Services – At Twice The Price You Are Now"
www.PaulsHiringBook.com

The Healthy Habit:
"Learn Secrets To Keep Active, Maintain Independence And Live Free From Painkillers. Essential Reading For People Aged 50+"
www.PaulsHealthyHabit.com

Printed in Great Britain
by Amazon